FUEL THE FIRE

FUEL

A NUTRITION AND BODY

THE FIRE

CONFIDENCE GUIDEBOOK FOR THE FEMALE ATHLETE

PAMELA NISEVICH BEDE, MS, RD

AVERY

AVERY

an imprint of Penguin Random House LLC
penguinrandomhouse.com

Most Avery books are available at special quantity discounts for bulk purchase for sales promotions, premiums, fund-raising, and educational needs. Special books or book excerpts also can be created to fit specific needs. For details, write: SpecialMarkets@penguinrandomhouse.com.

Library of Congress Cataloging-in-Publication Data

Names: Bede, Pamela Nisevich, author.
Title: Fuel the fire: a nutrition and body confidence guidebook for the female athlete / by Pamela Nisevich Bede, MS, RD.
Description: [New York]: Avery, [2022] | Includes index.
Identifiers: LCCN 2022003299 (print) | LCCN 2022003300 (ebook) | ISBN 9780593418642 (Trade Paperback) | ISBN 9780593418659 (ePub)
Subjects: LCSH: Women athletes—Training of. | Sports for women—Physiological aspects. | Physical fitness for women.
Classification: LCC GV709.B43 2022 (print) | LCC GV709 (ebook) | DDC 796.082—dc23/eng/20220408
LC record available at https://lccn.loc.gov/2022003299
LC ebook record available at https://lccn.loc.gov/2022003300

Printed in the United States of America
1st Printing

Book design by Laura K. Corless

To Miller, Hunter, and Piper:
Always let your little light shine

CONTENTS

PART 3
THIS GIRL IS ON FIRE

FUEL THE FIRE

PART 1

COLLECT THE KINDLING

THE PATH FORWARD:
A FEW NOTES FROM THE EXPERT

WHY THIS BOOK MATTERS

My kids often ask me, "Mom, can I really be anything I want to be?" Like any parent offering the company line, I respond with "Yes, anything is possible." But the pragmatist in me adds a caveat. You can be anything if you're willing to work for it. You'll need endless dedication, grit, proper fuel, a bit of luck (it also helps if the genetic gods smile on you), and the right support to get you there.

But here's the thing. Somewhere between the bliss of childhood and the realities of adulthood, we come to learn that there's a real world out there. And the real world is hard. It often feels as if the critics outnumber the fans. And depending on the relevant influences, the thickness of our skin, and our support systems, we can find our trajectory changed—for better or for worse.

Knowing this, I want to tell them: "I know you can set the world on fire, but I can't tell you exactly how." I can't tell you the exact path to the peak of a mountain, but I do know you won't get there without working for it. And I can show you several paths that will NOT take you to the top, because I've followed some of these paths. These are frustrating and a waste of time or dark and desolate and lead you in the wrong direction.

And that's why this book matters. The knowledge shared in these pages, along with the aid of experts, leaders, and mentors, will help you find your best self. So whether you're currently on the right road and just need a few directions or you are so lost you feel like you might never get where you want to go, you've got help here. No matter where you are on your nutrition journey, you're not alone in your desire to build a better relationship with food and self or to finally find a better way to meet your health, lifestyle, and performance goals. Soon you'll begin to see that light at the end of the tunnel, provided by someone who went before you and took the time to look back and weigh in with real-world advice and insights across the pages of this book.

WHO IS THIS BOOK FOR?

Fitness enthusiasts, competitors, contenders, Olympians, elites, age-group stars, rising stars, mother runners, anyone too busy putting in the work to do much grandstanding.

I wrote this book for those who exercise with purpose. For sweaty people familiar with terms like *Dri-FIT* and *fartlek* and *gels*. For those who link their identity with action verbs. For those who own multiple pairs of running shoes. For those who see opportunities to race when they look at their calendar and feel a bit lost when not actively pursuing one goal or another. Those dedicated to the cause and the process rather than winning at all costs. Who realize life is you versus you, and therefore you are your biggest critic or your biggest fan. This book is for those who have not yet learned that life is more marathon than sprint and for those who could teach a course on that exact lesson. For those who haven't even peaked and those trying their damnedest to reignite a lost spark.

Am I speaking your language? Then get ready to learn what it takes to build your best self yet. Ounce by ounce, cell by cell, built by better nutrition, habits, perspectives.

Find Pro Tips and strategies that are rooted in science and supported by practice. Advice shared while fueling countless athletes and friends throughout my time as a sports dietitian, mom, and athlete. And advice from elite athletes, coaches, Olympians, scientists, and leaders weighing in on lessons learned across their own nutrition journeys.

Discover how to rock game-day fueling, eat for health, and tear down obstacles in your path. Most of all, I hope you evolve to be comfortable in your own skin and build an amazing relationship with food. I'm here to teach you how to develop a way of eating that fuels and sustains. It's now more important than ever to uncover a way to prevent and fix muddied, broken relationships with food and self. Once you are no longer willing to listen to misinformation or give way to negativity, this book will become your weapon in the fight against internal doubts and external critics.

So from the track to the road to the pitch to the gym, classroom to internship to office to home, you'll build a nutrition foundation that's so solid, it will support you as you crank out countless miles and endless training sessions, and then recover and ultimately thrive. Get ready to fill a plate that works for YOU. To finally understand what it takes to fuel *your* performance, *your* health, and *your* best self.

DEAR YOUNGER, HUNGRY ME

What if you could go back in time and offer advice to your younger self? What would you say? How would you mentor the younger you? How would you respond to the countless important questions? Questions about whether your dedication to sport was worth it. Questions about what you should eat and why these choices were important. Questions about how to navigate dark days, work through relationships, and avoid obstacles.

Each of us has a journey to share, insights to impart. We can't change the past, but we can learn from it. The letters that flow across these pages are here to help you build a better future based on knowledge gleaned from the past.

DEAR YOUNGER, HUNGRY ME: JOAN BENOIT SAMUELSON

Joan Benoit Samuelson could be described as the godmother of women's running. She's a venerated world record holder, a gold medal Olympian, a course record holder, and winner of several prestigious road races, including the first women's Olympic Marathon, the Chicago Marathon, the Falmouth Road Race (six times), and the Beach to Beacon 10K (a race she founded). In 2019, she ran the Boston Marathon, forty years after her 1979 win, with a goal of finishing within forty minutes of her winning time. She did even better. With a wicked fast time of 3:04:00, she crossed the finish within 30 minutes of her previous time, winning her age group (sixty to sixty-four) along the way.

Those close to Joan describe her as a humble, gracious, determined runner from Maine who loves the outdoors, her garden, and skiing. She's unquestionably a passionate advocate for the sport of running. Spend time with Joan and you're bound to meet someone whose life she's changed for the better. She's unknowingly inspired complete strangers to pick up a pair of running shoes, start putting one foot in front of the other, and become a better version of themselves. Along the way, Joan has shattered glass ceilings, shown countless women what is possible, and served as an exemplar for balancing motherhood and work. She humorously divides her career into two distinct phases: Before Children and After Diapers. Joan is honest, kind, and real. I'm honored to call her friend and elated to share her letter with you.

Dear Younger, Hungry Joan,

Your growing passion for running is about to open some amazing doors of opportunity. Your talent will lead you through, and the result will help others understand all that can be possible when you pursue your dreams. As you chase these dreams, always listen to your heart and your gut too. Remember, you have nothing to prove except to yourself.

As you mature, listen to the wisdom of those who matter: your parents, teachers, coaches, and friends. But don't underestimate the value of your own opinion as well. Don't be afraid to dream too big, because while there will continue to be a lack of opportunities, as a young girl and woman you can start the wheels of change. The women who have gone before you have begun to pave the way, and now you get to help define what is possible and then redefine it for yourself and for other young women.

Protect your dreams, be willing to work for them, and never say never. Don't be afraid of setting lofty goals; should you fail, you'll be a stronger person for it. Do not compromise; set intermediate stepping-stones until you reach what's possible. Otherwise, you will be cutting your true potential short. The first women's Olympic Marathon? A lofty goal that will help you and the world understand what's possible.

You will look for opportunities that will benefit others and you will benefit as well. Your neighborhood community of friends—not boys, not girls, just children—will include you and push you. They will make you feel welcome in their games and activities, and you'll become stronger as a result of trying to keep up with their physical activities. Remember to play hard with passion and consideration. These early days and friends are valuable, setting the foundation for what it means to be an integral part of a family, team, and community. That makes you who you are. Push your limits as an individual, but embrace the old adage "There is no I in team."

Remember to be kind and empathetic to those whom you meet as you mature. When it comes to fueling your body and spirit, don't forget the importance that parents put on being there physically and mentally at mealtime. Mother will serve nourishing, well-balanced meals by making meals colorful. You will continue to thrive on local and fresh garden-rich offerings. Soda and candy will be treats and not readily available (except when visiting grandmother)! Look for the hidden gumdrops and jelly beans she'll hide while she babysits and everyone naps. Hold this memory tight. And let this be an early education regarding treats and rewards.

Always believe that there is no finish line to possibility and potential.

Believe in yourself. Live by the old proverb "If at first you don't succeed, try, try again." There are no shortcuts to hard work, but it's a lot easier if there is passion.

Sincerely,

Joan

WHY NUTRITION MATTERS

If you're searching for that one person who can change your life for the better, go find a mirror.

Nutrition is a science, but eating involves emotion. And given that we're more often emotional than rational when it comes to food, it can be hard to act on nutritional tactics that we all know work. We ourselves, including what we eat, change constantly, fluctuating with the stage of life we're in and with the passing seasons, often in response to needing to deal with whatever our day hands us. There's nothing wrong with changing: after all, our bodies, including our physical and health needs, change, and our nutrition must change in order for us to adapt and rise to the occasion. But when our diet changes for the worse, not for the better, it's time to take note.

We naturally mature from eating for survival to eating with purpose and for wellness and pleasure. But as emotional beings, we can easily become overwhelmed by appetite, a dizzying array of options, and the criticism of others, coping by eating too much or not at all. For some, there is no in-between. And the solace and support we once received from gatherings around the dinner table with family, friends, and teammates can disappear, replaced by hectic schedules, takeout, distrust, and outside influencers pushing their own notion of "the perfect plate."

It's a jungle out there. The stress that surrounds food threatens our relationship with the very sustenance that enables us to survive.

If you're like most, you've got a handle on what purposeful nutrition looks like. Consistently translating that knowledge into action, however, is a struggle. Or perhaps you find that your body is objecting to the foods you're eating. Or what works one day of the month falls flat a week later. Or you rock at eating healthy when you're in a good mindset but get totally derailed anytime you're injured or stressed. We'll explore tactics to help you build better habits and employ female-forward science to build a plan as unique as you. And if you're struggling with energy availability or restricting what's on your plate, we'll explore ways to recover.

Today's lifestyle can shake even the strongest of nutritional foundations. Even the relatively confident and well-informed are inundated with conflicting research, unfounded advice, and *plenty* of unsolicited opinions on what to eat. Welcome to a world where the majority of us no longer feel confident in our food choices or our own skin.

TIME FOR A CHANGE

Enough is enough. It's time to better understand the real science of nutrition and the elements of female physiology and female health so we can own our plate, fuel ourselves to support the fire within, and ultimately rebuild a better relationship with food.

In the effort to become your best, healthiest, most powerful self, finding the right fuel matters. Eating with purpose in mind, consuming the optimal fuel in the right amounts at the right time and even on the right day of the month will help you feel energized and nourished rather than fatigued, injured, or ill. If you gain an understanding of basic nutrition and the best sources of nutrients and learn how to navigate dining halls, own your kitchen, or meal prep and plan like a pro, you'll be on the right path.

If you're ready to help create a world in which better nutrition and better image of self can thrive, I'm glad you're here. If you're determined to find fuel that works for *you*—fuel that responds to the needs of your unique female physiology—and to fight back against outdated advice, unfounded opinions, and negativity, this guidebook is for you. Let's start learning how to love and nourish the skin we're in, challenge our expectations of ourselves, enhance our performance, and fuel the fire for the weeks, months, and years to come.

MAPPING OUT DAILY ENERGY NEEDS

At times, when I introduce myself as a dietitian, I end up regretting I've said anything. I'm inevitably peppered with overly personal questions about nutrition, leaving me to wonder, once again, why I didn't lie and say I sell appliances. Strangers consistently ask me how many calories they should eat. I'm certain a look of disbelief floods my face when I hear this question, as the supposedly simple task of calculating calorie needs is anything but.

Many of our nutritional concerns revolve around the humble calorie, because this ubiquitous unit of energy holds a lot of sway. The power to fuel our day. The power to fuel miles and speed. Not enough calories and we hit the wall or crumble. Too many and we need to nap or go shopping for a bigger pair of pants.

Determining your calorie needs is just one step in figuring out your perfect plate, and if you skip this step, you can still navigate toward health and performance. Because honestly, the makeup of your plate—the nutritional quality or nutrient density of chosen foods—is much more important than the number of calories it contains. Countless factors impact your caloric requirements, given that your caloric needs vary from day to day—depending on how much and how intensely you're training and what point you're at in your training cycle—and across the stages of your life. The number of calories you need today will not be the same as you need tomorrow and in the future.

For some, establishing a calorie goal is unnecessary and potentially dangerous. It can take you to a dark place if you're predisposed to let hitting this number derail your day or if you tend to equate calories with self-worth. Don't give it that power.

In my practice, I often find that identifying a calorie *range* can be valuable in keeping you supplied with the energy you need to support optimal body function, in helping you determine how much of each macronutrient to consume, and in bringing you one step closer to your body composition goals.

DRIVERS OF ENERGY NEEDS

Your body requires energy all the time to keep it fully functioning. Add in activity and this energy demand increases. The unit of energy that food provides is the simple calorie. The following factors determine the number of calories you need to feel your best and perform at the top of your game:

- Your basal metabolic rate (BMR)—the energy needed to keep your systems functioning while at rest
- The thermic effect of food (TEF)—the energy needed to digest food
- The thermic effect of activity (TEA)—the energy needed to move and composed of multiple factors:
  a. Spontaneous physical activity—physical behavior that emanates from an unconscious drive for movement (e.g., fidgeting)
  b. Exercise—a range of demanding behaviors, varying across seasons and training blocks
  c. Non-exercise activity thermogenesis—energy expended for everything we do that is not sleeping, eating, or sports-like exercise

For sedentary individuals, the basal metabolic rate accounts for 60 to 80 percent of daily calorie needs, while in active individuals, BMR accounts for much less—as little as 38 to 47 percent of energy expenditure. TEF accounts for 10 percent of energy expenditure, and the components of TEA account for the remainder. If we take into account training loads and activities of daily life, TEA can range from minimal impact in sedentary populations to over 50 percent of total energy expenditure in athletes.

For athletes, some factors have the potential to increase—to varying degrees—caloric needs above baseline requirements. These factors include:

- Exposure to cold or heat
- Fear and stress
- High-altitude training
- Various injuries
- Specific drugs or medications
- The luteal phase of the menstrual cycle

For athletes, factors with the potential to decrease caloric needs above baseline requirements include:

- Reductions in training
- Aging
- Decreases in fat-free mass
- The follicular phase of the menstrual cycle

Pro Tip: *Tempted to use an online calculator or app to determine optimal calorie needs? Proceed with caution. Most often these tools ask for very few inputs— gender, weight (or goal weight), age—and generally result in a wholly inaccurate representation of an athlete's true energy needs. Make sure the tool you use asks for multiple inputs, and if the calculator kicks out a recommendation that is less than 1,500 calories a day, it's probably not taking into account the energy needed for your stage of life, training, performance, and health.*

TEST WISELY

Without a doubt, the best way to determine your energy needs is in a lab setting, using a dual-energy X-ray absorptiometry (DEXA or DXA) scan to measure body composition, plus an indirect calorimetry machine for resting metabolic rate measurements. A variety of testing methods are usually available (see page 31) at university nutrition clinics or exercise physiology labs (so ask around if you're a collegiate athlete). The rest of us can gain access to these precise measurements via a hospital lab setting or a sports medicine clinic, or simply through a local university. Consider making an appointment and getting scanned so you know the state of your bone health as well as how much of your mass is lean tissue and how much is fat mass. Consider having your BMR tested rather than estimated; more precise data allows for a more confident approach when mapping out a fueling plan.

When gold-standard DEXAs and lab-based tests are not readily available, we use other tools (that is to say, math) in a clinic setting and on the sidelines. Validated equations like the one listed on the following page are often relied upon to estimate your daily caloric needs. Remember, these equations offer merely a starting point, a goal that will evolve over time, just like you. So grab a pencil and a calculator and let's get started.

LET'S TALK ABOUT WEIGHT

Keep in mind that the number on the scale is just one element to consider when you are thinking about your health and athletic performance. Your current weight does serve as a starting point and is a required factor in metabolism equations. But before you get to adding and subtracting, pause to consider where you are and where you'd like to be. Is your current weight healthy? Is your goal weight realistic? To answer these questions for clients, I consider more than just one number; I take into account the person's body mass index, ideal body weight, and feel-good weight.

Body Mass Index: What Is It?

Your body mass index, or BMI, is a ratio of weight to height calculated by dividing your weight (in kilograms) by your height (in meters, squared). This screening tool is often used as an indicator of obesity and underweight but is not used to diagnose body composition or health. The calculation of a body mass index has significant limitations, such as overestimating body fat in muscular athletes and underestimating body fat in those who have lost muscle mass. For example, I've seen a number of "overweight" young athletes who are in excellent health with strong, lean physiques and who can run a sub-6-minute mile. I've also seen a lot of "healthy weight" athletes who desperately need more muscle mass to support their sport or who are deficient in nutrient intake and battling a disordered approach to eating.

BMI is rarely a priority metric for athletes, but it can prove useful in setting a baseline weight status for those in the general population. BMI is also a good gauge of risk for diseases that tend to develop as your percentage of body fat increases, underlining why you're likely to hear your health care professional use this term. Higher BMIs can be correlated with higher risk of certain diseases such as heart disease, high blood pressure, type 2 diabetes, gallstones, breathing problems, and certain cancers. BMIs categorized as underweight correlate with health risks such as a weakened immune system, malnutrition, poor bone health, and lower muscle mass.

Body Mass Index: Calculate It

Your body mass index is calculated by dividing your weight in kilograms by your height in square meters (kg/m^2). If you prefer American measurements, the equation for BMI is:

Weight in pounds × 703 / (Height in inches × Height in inches)
Calculate your BMI: _____

Another, simpler alternative is just to go to a reliable online BMI calculator and plug in your weight and height. You'll find one at https://www.cdc.gov/healthyweight/assessing /bmi/adult_bmi/english_bmi_calculator/bmi_calculator.html.

Now, what does that mean? Are you at a healthy BMI or should you consider striving for a lower number, one better for your health? Or is your BMI low and could you be heading toward injury and illness as you drop further into the underweight category?

BMI is classified into underweight, healthy weight, overweight, and obese.The categories are as follows:

Underweight = less than 18.5
Healthy weight = 18.5 to less than 25
Overweight = 25 to less than 30
Obese = 30 or higher

Ideal Body Weight: What Is It?

Now, let's consider your ideal body weight using the Hammond Method:

Simplistically defined, ideal body weight (IBW) is a term used to indicate a target body weight for nutritional and health assessments. IBW equations (and quite a few exist) are formulated to predict weight as a linear function of height, so you can see that this metric doesn't necessarily take form and fitness level or stage of life wholly into the equation. Fairly straightforward to calculate, IBW, much like BMI, should be taken with a grain of salt. To begin with, IBW was originally defined as the weight associated with the greatest life expectancy at each height, but there is no single ideal weight that applies universally to all health conditions and all demographics. On paper, IBW equations may yield a specific body weight, but in reality, nutrition experts and clinical data support a *range* of target body weights. Finally, researchers have analyzed IBW equations and showed that IBW equations tend to underestimate body weight at shorter heights and overestimate body weights at taller heights. In most settings, IBW equations have largely been replaced by BMI ranges. But for purposes of this discussion, you can determine your ideal body weight using the Hammond equation, which is frequently used for nutrition assessments. I recommend adding +/–10 percent to arrive at a range.

Ideal Body Weight: Calculate It

Female: Wt** (kg) = 45 + 0.9 × (Ht* − 150 cm) +/−10%

Male: Wt** (kg) = 48 + 1.1 × (Ht* − 150 cm) +/−10%

*Height in centimeters. Convert height in inches to centimeters by
   multiplying by 2.54.

**Weight in kilograms. Convert weight in pounds to kilograms by dividing by 2.2.

For example, the ideal body weight of a 5'5" female would be calculated as:

5'5" = 65 inches = 165.1 cm

[45 + 0.9 × (165.1 − 150)] +/−10%

[45 + 0.9 × (15.1)] +/−10% = 58.6 kg +/−10% → 52.7 to 64.5 kg

Convert kilograms to pounds by multiplying by 2.2. Thus, in pounds,
   IBW = 129 lb +/−10%, or a range of 116 to 142 pounds.

Using Body Composition to Identify a More Precise Ideal Body Weight

The human body is made up of lean mass, fat mass, and a host of other factors (like water). General equations can't get to the root of what you're made of. But if you have data in hand following a DEXA scan or other vetted method, you can assess if you're where you *want* to be. Note I didn't say determine if you're where your coach wants you to be or where you *need* to be. Remember, nothing supports the idea that body fat percentage of X percent equals X minutes per mile or X place on the podium. (To learn more about the measurement and impact of body composition, see pages 29–34). Body composition is one factor out of many, so you'd be better off spending time planning a better plate, understanding nutrient timing, or strengthening your core rather than chasing a specific ratio of fat mass to lean mass.

Still, this metric proves useful to many. Let's say you have your body composition checked and you learn that 22 percent of your 5'5", 130-pound female body is fat mass. This is well within normal, healthy limits, but you feel that with some simple dietary changes, you could shed some fat mass while still feeling energized and perhaps improving your performance. You target a 10 percent reduction, down from 22 to 20 percent body fat, and will monitor yourself to see if you feel lighter and more powerful. So how to determine the IBW to get you there?

STEP 1: Determine current percentage of fat mass and lean mass as well as goal percentages.
Current: 22% body fat, 78% lean
Goal: 20% body fat, 80% lean

STEP 2: Calculate lean body mass (lb).
Lean body mass = your lean body mass percentage at your current weight
130 lb × 78% lean (0.78) = 101 lb of lean muscle mass (that you don't want to shed)

STEP 3: Determine estimated ideal body weight.
Divide lean body mass by optimal lean body mass percentage
101 lb / 80% (0.80) = 126 lb

Checks and Balances Matter

The motivation to reach an ideal body weight or a goal weight varies from person to person. But in athletes, the motivation is almost always rooted in performance. Athletes are wired to do what it takes to improve, whether that's train harder, take recovery seriously, skip happy hour, or lose excess weight. But when we identify what we perceive to be an excess of body weight and decide to take ideal body weight to extremes, the above equation can begin to spiral out of control.

Using the athlete in the example on the previous page, a shift from current 22 percent body fat down to an arbitrary 8 percent body fat might spark hope of improved performance. Ignore the fact that a female athlete with only 8 percent body fat is dipping into essential stores needed to support physiological functions, not to mention that arriving at this low number and staying at it for a while will likely bring about health complications. If we use that equation, 8 percent body fat would equate to an ideal body weight of less than 110 pounds. According to the Hammond equation, at this weight a 5'5" female athlete is well outside the range of healthy or athletic. A weight loss this great would result in a BMI of 18.3kg/m², or clinically underweight.

There are checks and balances when it comes to determining a weight that will work to support your health and performance goals, so use more than one tool to find a range that can work for you.

Find Your Feel-Good Weight

One such tool that I use with athletes is what I call your feel-good weight. That is, rather than focusing on some magical and elusive weight, try asking yourself: *At what weight do*

> **Pro Tip:** Let's talk about race weight. I can't overemphasize the fact that while assessment and manipulation of body composition can better one's performance, taken to extremes this manipulation does the exact opposite. For some, healthy reductions in weight may improve performance. But left unchecked, continued reductions will result in a breaking point. While there is an undeniable connection between body weight and performance, athletic performance can't be predicted or guaranteed based on body composition or a number on the scale. Let that sink in. The mere fact that you hit a number on the scale does not assure you a place on the podium. And conversely, if you fail to hit race weight before the big day, this doesn't mean you won't win. Spending lots of time and energy chasing some arbitrary number is both unproductive and unhealthy.

I feel good? This means that you feel full of energy and ready to tackle your day, and your blood pressure, heart rate, blood glucose, and blood lipid levels are right where your doctor wants them to be. When you arrive at this number, compare it to your ideal body weight range, aim to fall within a healthy BMI, and you'll have a great place to start.

FIGHTING THAT FEELING OF "FAT"

Let's address the uncomfortable subject of the number on the scale. Because determining what your "ideal" weight is, listening to what someone else deems a desirable weight, or simply considering your actual body weight can increase conversations around feelings of "fatness." The vast majority of college-age women and about a quarter of college-age males commiserate over feeling fat, yet few are actually overweight.

Peer-to-peer chats may be extremely common among women and men, but they aren't productive. And while we all look for empathy or reassurance, Simon Marshall, PhD, coauthor of *The Brave Athlete*, says these conversations aren't moving us in the right direction. Marshall notes that while women believe "fat talk" makes them feel better, the opposite happens. Such conversations often leave us feeling even more dissatisfied with our bodies. And evolving research suggests that these sisterhood confession sessions can actually contribute to weight gain: they add psychological stress and lead to unsustainable dietary habits that contribute to weight gain. What you thought was a cathartic discussion is usually destructive. So skip the fat talk.

Marshall suggests when you "feel" fat, this can be a smoke screen for other feelings: frustration over a training session gone wrong or a lack of control over food habits; jealousy over someone's genetic predisposition to be built a certain way. You see where this is going.

When you experience a feeling of fatness, pause to consider what might have triggered it. In this case, a trigger is a circumstance or event that prompted you to respond in a certain way. Sort through the underlying emotions and ask yourself if there's a pattern to the times you feel fat. Are there certain triggers or environments or even people who continue to lead you to this state of dissatisfaction with your body?

Remember, it's normal to feel fat occasionally, and depending on the day of the month and the fuel in your tank; remember that your weight does indeed fluctuate. Your long-term goal is to be aware that your body is dynamic, and thus these feelings happen. Acknowledge them but don't react to them. Don't let feelings of fatness own your day. You're too strong for that. Move on.

If you're really struggling to navigate your way around negative feelings about yourself or about food, or if these internal conversations seem to be happening more and more, it may be time to ask for help.

DETERMINING CALORIE NEEDS

Start with determining your basal metabolic rate (BMR), the bare minimum number of calories you need each day to keep your vital organs functioning—your brain thinking, your heart pumping, and so on. Calculate this number based on your weight today. (We'll discuss the necessary math for making changes to your weight in a bit.) BMR is typically not a high number because it represents the number of calories your body needs at rest.

Here's how to determine your basal metabolic rate using the Mifflin-St. Jeor equation:

1. Start with your weight in kilograms: just divide your weight in pounds by 2.2.

2. Next, convert your height to centimeters: multiply your height in inches by 2.54.

3. Now, apply this formula:
   Female: [10 × weight (kg)] + [6.25 × height (cm)] − [5 × age (yr)] − 161 = _____
   Male: [10 × weight (kg)] + [6.25 × height (cm)] − [5 × age (yr)] + 5 = _____

The resulting number is your estimated basal metabolic rate. Remember, this is the amount of energy needed to fuel a day in bed (which sounds lovely, BTW). To fuel your day-to-day activities and performance, multiply this number by a physical activity level (PAL) factor (more on that in a bit).

Note: Many online BMR calculators use the Harris-Benedict equation to determine BMR. For athletes, many practitioners use the Mifflin-St. Jeor to more accurately estimate needs.

> **Pro Tip:** In sedentary individuals, BMR (energy needs while resting) represents about 60 to 80 percent of total energy expenditure. You're not sedentary. Instead, there's a wide range of calories to consider adding to BMR in order to adequately fuel your day. And this number could be significant: research finds that BMR may account for less than 34 to 42 percent of total daily needs in elite endurance athletes.

MAINTAINING WEIGHT AND PERFORMANCE

Whether your current weight matches your goal weight or not, accurately accounting for both BMR and level of physical activity is critical to identifying the amount of energy you need throughout the day. The more active you are, the more energy you need to consume to support your athletic performance and crank through your workouts, even if weight loss is a goal. Think of it this way. Let's say you pre-fuel with a 150-calorie snack and then run 5 miles, burning an estimated 500 calories. Exercise burn minus pre-exercise fuel equals a caloric deficit of 350 calories. Now let's say you skipped the pre-workout fuel and struggled to cover the distance, stopping short at 3 miles. You created a deficit of 300 calories. Adding a little bit of fuel can support your performance and the metabolic adaptations that come with exercise while also allowing you to create a bigger deficit. So don't skimp when it comes to fueling your activity.

To determine how much energy you need to support health and sport, you'll identify your physical activity level (PAL) factor and multiply by your BMR. PALs were established by the Institute of Medicine to determine the amount of energy expended across bouts of physical activity. PALs are most accurate for sedentary individuals because energy expended during workouts varies greatly from day to day, session to session. Identify your PAL factor using the "Ask Yourself" questions in the chart on the following page.

Choose a range of PAL that best suits your day. Your training load shifts from day to day, so your PAL factor will change daily as well. Thus your calorie needs will be greater on days slated for heavy training than on recovery days. In my clinical practice, when I'm estimating calorie needs for weight loss, maintenance, and weight gain, I narrowly define ranges using varying PALs. I find this more precise than adding or subtracting some arbitrary number of calories from a BMR.

WHICH PAL IS RIGHT FOR YOU?

That depends on your goals. If weight loss will improve your performance, you might target the low end of the PAL range. Those interested in weight maintenance should choose a midrange PAL, and those striving for increases in body mass can consult the upper end of the range. As always, these ranges and outputs are simply an estimate. There is substantial room for error for athletes based on the significant energy cost of exercise on some days and not on others. Listen to your body, considering your levels of fatigue and hunger and your ability to recover. Don't let a number steer you toward low energy availability or the related relative energy deficiency in sport (RED-S), which will be discussed in greater depth on page 224.

DETERMINE YOUR PAL

Physical Activity Level Category	Ask Yourself	Low End (weight loss)	Midrange (weight maintenance)	High End (weight gain)
SEDENTARY	Do you spend most of your day resting, sitting, studying?	1.1	1.25	1.39
LOW	Are you up and about during the day but don't participate in purposeful physical activity? Are you temporarily sedentary due to recovering from an injury?	1.4	1.5	1.59
LIGHTLY ACTIVE	Do you exercise 30 minutes a day or walk the equivalent of 6 miles a day?	1.6	1.7	1.8
MODERATELY ACTIVE	Do you exercise an hour a day or walk the equivalent of 8-plus miles a day?	1.7	1.8	1.9
HIGHLY ACTIVE	Are you intensely training for a race or competition, exercising 2 to 3 hours a day?	1.9	2.2	2.5

Example: A thirty-year-old woman weighs 140 pounds. She is 5'6" and has determined that with some nutritional improvements, she can get a bit faster and leaner. She works out 30 minutes every day and wants to reach 130 lbs, which, based on BMI and IBW equations, is within a healthy range.

Weight: 140 lb / 2.2 = 63.6 kg

Height: 5'6" → 66 in × 2.54 = 167.6 cm

$[[10 \times 63.6] + [6.25 \times 167.6] - [5 \times 30] - 161] \times$ PAL factor of 1.6

$[[636] + [1047.5] - [150] - 161] \times 1.6 = 2{,}196$ calories needed to support activity and facilitate weight loss

As you can see, determining calorie needs is not as simple as doing mental math on the fly. Now that you have a range to help you ID your daily energy needs, you can get started mapping out a plan for your daily macronutrient intake. Remember, what's more important than total calorie intake is calorie value. In fact, some people never track caloric intake, instead focusing on making healthy, whole food choices.

If you choose to calculate calories, consider this metric as a helpful guide while you build your best plate, incorporating colorful, nutrient-dense foods to fuel you. Use it to determine how to divvy up your calories so that you consume adequate carbohydrate, protein, and fat.

Hitting or missing a target caloric intake in a given day is not essential, and if you find yourself obsessing over numbers, avoid calculating this metric. But if you find that having a target number to aim toward is helpful in keeping you on track, you now have this tool in your toolbox. Remember to check back in on your energy needs estimate every now and then, since it can change over time.

THE INTRICACIES OF BODY COMPOSITION

You've now mapped out your calorie needs, understanding that the math represents just one point in time and that your needs change day to day, influenced by a host of factors. The number you arrived at should be adequate to support your day-to-day energy needs and your physical structure—your weight and body composition. Keep in mind that there is no perfect weight. And while there are ranges to consider, there's no perfect body composition, either.

At its core, body composition consists of lean mass and fat mass. You need proper portions of each to hit your health goals, and different sports often call for different body compositions.

Lean mass is composed of metabolically active tissue: organs, bone, muscle.
Fat mass is made up of adipose tissue and other lipid storage.

Should *you* decide you want to make improvements to body composition, like trading fat tissue for lean tissue or adding more muscle to power your workout and longevity, such targeted improvements can add more value than simply hitting a random number on the scale. Such improvements often occur over time in a natural fashion through changes in nutrition and increases in training. Modifications of your body composition can have a greater impact than gains or losses of weight because what you're made of matters. Lose too much fat mass and you'll become malnourished and fatigued, and you may have irregular periods or stop menstruating. Lose too much lean mass and you'll shed the muscle needed to power you, and the bone density needed to support you.

BAPTIZED ON BODY COMPOSITION

When it comes to performance and sport, body composition is simply one spoke on the wheel of performance. We're often guilty of giving body composition more credit in bettering our performance than it truly deserves. It's not always our fault—we live in a world that values appearance. Also, whether we realize it or not, we often gravitate toward sports that favor our current or potential body type, hoping for success based on some ingrained belief that composition drives excellence. Sometimes this feels like a form of natural selection, but often choices are dictated by parents, who will sign their offspring up for a sport with exclamations of "You'd be so good at this!" or will discourage their children from an activity with "You want to try what? Are you sure?"

Whether we like it or not, our physical makeup has some impact on our success in a specific sport. But such success depends upon a variety of things, each with varying degrees of impact. When we're talking about body composition, this impact ranges from superior athletic prowess to superior aesthetics. Athletes in aesthetically oriented sports—dance, gymnastics, figure skating, and diving, for example—may believe they will be judged or scored more favorably if they have a lean body build. Often their beliefs are not unfounded. Success in gravitational sports is primarily dictated by physics. Distance runners and cyclists fight gravity with each step and pedal stroke; to a degree, less weight allows for more efficient acceleration and less drag. Athletes in weight-class sports—for example, wrestling and martial arts—deliberately tinker with their weight in order to compete in a specific weight class—typically the lowest achievable. Athletes in sports such as football and bodybuilding work toward a heavy and muscular physique, while start-and-stop sports such as soccer and lacrosse, which call for speed and agility, draw on those with a lean, mean, and muscular body build.

Sports That Favor a Lean Physique (gravitational and aesthetic)	Sports That Favor a Muscular Build	Weight-Class Sports
Dance and cheerleading	Basketball	Boxing
Running	Bodybuilding	Crew
Figure skating	CrossFit	Martial arts
Cycling	Football and rugby	Wrestling
Swimming (synchronized or racing) and diving	Lacrosse	Combat sports
Gymnastics	Soccer	Horse racing
Skiing	Track: throwing (discus, javelin, shot put)	Weight lifting

HOW TO TEST: MEASURING BODY COMPOSITION

There are several methods of measuring body fat percentage, and depending upon the method used, there is often a margin of error to consider. Dual-energy X-ray absorptiometry (DEXA or DXA), air displacement plethysmography (e.g., the Bod Pod), underwater weighing, skinfold measurements, and bioelectrical impedance analysis (BIA) are all common methods for ascertaining one's body composition. DEXA is a scanning technique that accurately estimates bone mineral, fat, and lean tissue. It is considered the gold standard, but the test is involved and can be expensive. DEXA is becoming more readily accessible; most university sports medicine departments and many hospitals have the ability to run this test. BIA is the method you'll encounter when using a home scale that includes a body fat percentage reading (these are typically the scales with metal plates placed where your heel and forefoot make contact). BIA readings are not always reliable and can be influenced by device calibration and accuracy as well as your hydration status. If you're using this method, consider it to be a baseline and observe general trends rather than putting significant value on the actual number. As for how often to test, athletes (and coaches or practitioners) who utilize body composition results typically check at the beginning of a season or block of training and then update their findings in three or six months.

WHAT TO LOOK FOR: BODY COMPOSITION RANGES

In healthy adults, body composition is typically consistent over the short term. The main determinants of your body composition are your gender, age, ethnicity, nutritional intake, physical activity habits, and hormonal status. While several factors influence your body composition, most of them are outside of your control. Your genes have a large influence. For example, if your parents are naturally lean, you likely will find a lower fat mass easier to achieve. But don't be discouraged if your genes aren't exactly what you'd choose or if you have a hard time shedding fat mass or really struggle to put on muscle mass. A third of the factors influencing your body composition are well within your control. Don't discount the power of nutrition and physical activity and other lifestyle choices to drive significant changes in the makeup of your body.

A thorough understanding and analysis of your body composition can be helpful *if* it gives you something positive to focus on—the building of lean muscle mass. If you take this approach, regardless of the number on the scale, you'll receive positive feedback as fat is replaced by lean muscle.

The body composition that is right for you depends on your athletic goals and your starting point. This is a situation in which you control what you can and realize that lower is not always better. Women in general need more essential fat stores than men in order to support their physiological functions and ensure their reproductive health. Female athletes naturally carry a higher percentage of fat mass compared to male athletes. Across the general population, reported body fat percentages and recommendations vary widely, but in general, women range from approximately 14 to 30 percent fat mass and men range from approximately 6 to 25 percent fat mass. Some research, albeit limited, has been done concerning ideal fat mass percentages for athletes in specific sports. Body fat percentages beyond either end of the spectrum carry significant negative health consequences.

BODY FAT RANGES FOR HEALTH AND PERFORMANCE

	Women	Men
ESSENTIAL FAT NEEDS	10-13%	2-5%
ATHLETES	12-21%	6-13%
GENERAL FITNESS	21-24%	14-17%
GENERAL HEALTH	21-31%	14-24%
OBESE	>32%	>25%

If you believe that achieving a low percentage of body fat will automatically ensure high performance, you are wrong. Time and again, superstar athletes perform, win, hit PRs with bodies that fall outside these zones. One case in point is Olympic marathoner and 2018 Boston Marathon champion Desiree "Des" Linden. Des naturally carries a distribution of lean to fat mass that falls within a performance range but at one point in time was deemed to be outside the range that some "experts" might consider indispensable to elite endurance performance. But what's missing from a number on paper is drive and determination, as well as the ability to come from behind and withstand frigid temperatures on a day when the Boston racecourse features torrential rains and hypothermic conditions. Classifying Des's potential based on a body composition report or assuming a race outcome dependent on whether an athlete has a traditional "runner's build" would be more than a grave mistake. It's insulting and erroneous.

Some athletes find that knowing their baseline, understanding their makeup, and making strides to improve an unhealthy ratio of fat to lean can be steps in the direction of health and performance. For others, having any such number in hand does more harm than good. Grayson Murphy, an all-American in cross-country and indoor and outdoor track, and now a world-class mountain runner, notes that throughout her collegiate career, body composition measurements via a Bod Pod were a mix of helpful, stressful, and hurtful. "It was helpful to see when my body fat percentage was too low for health." But when she was advised to put on weight to improve the metric, the weight she accrued was lean mass, therefore altering her percentage of body fat even further. Even when she was on the right track, the metric suggested she was failing. "As an intuitive person, I prefer to focus on how I feel versus a number. Measurements might be helpful to some, but they leave me feeling confused and misguided. My former team doesn't use Bod Pod measurements anymore."

CHASING A METRIC: A LONELY RACE?

Pursuing a specific body composition is not as prevalent as you might think. While you might hear a lot about percentages or be told that leaner absolutely equals faster, in the real world of competition, few elite teams and athletes are actually keeping track. And because this metric can be easily misconstrued, some teams don't allow such measurement. The University of Oregon recently announced that coaches may no longer subject athletes to body composition measurements, and if the athlete chooses to pursue a test, the results may not be reported beyond the student-athlete himself or herself and any relevant medical personnel or dietitians.

American long-distance runner Stephanie Bruce offered her opinion, noting that factors like sleep or mileage or fueling are much more important than body composition. Bruce can't remember when her body composition was tested last, doesn't track this likely unhelpful and potentially harmful metric, and cautioned that everyone's body composition is different. With a smile, she noted being beaten by runners who weighed more than she did and on paper looked less formidable. At the finish line, weight and body composition don't matter. What matters is who breaks the tape. Bruce never viewed losing as a result of weight or body composition. "If I got beat, I thought, *Maybe they work harder than me, or maybe they're simply more talented.* Performance is rarely centered on weight. You have to switch your mindset and then ask yourself: *Do* I *need to work harder? Am* I *working hard enough?*"

Bruce added that "if you've figured out every other part of racing and training and you're still not seeing the expected results, body composition might matter. Otherwise, performance is dependent on other, more powerful factors." So in Des's words, "Don't let the internet or any outsider dictate how you feel you need to look. The only right way is the one where you're healthy and confident." And, I might add, crushing the competition.

DEAR YOUNGER, HUNGRY ME: DES LINDEN

The race is the reward. On a frigid spring day complete with torrential rain and punishing hail, Des Linden captured the hearts of the world when she overcame unprecedented conditions. Her journey toward the winner's circle reflects much of her perspective on running. She moved from questioning her own ability to realizing "I can win this." She traversed the miles while sacrificing her own performance for the betterment of her friends. She selflessly helped other American runners bridge the gaps in the race. Ultimately, she herself prevailed, breaking the tape and becoming the first American female in thirty-three years to win the storied Boston Marathon. Her list of accomplishments includes representing the United States two times in the Olympic marathon and holding the 50K record, and she'll be the first to tell you that the path isn't always smooth. At some points along the way, you doubt yourself and your training. But past failures don't identify you—they provide you with an opportunity to grow. Des knows that sometimes performance just flows and sometimes sport puts us through hell. But every day you're handed a choice. And Des chooses to keep pursuing what's possible and making room for miracles, and ultimately she continues to show up.

Dear Younger, Hungry Des,

Grab a snack and let's chat. You've always held the view that food is functional, it's fuel for you to participate in sports. This was drilled into your mind at a young age and to some degree took the fun out of food, but it was an important lesson and stuck with you. Want to play sports? You must eat. Simple. From a nutritional point of view, there were plenty of missing lessons, but starting with the idea that something, even if it's the "wrong" thing, is better than nothing isn't the worst place to be.

Sticking with the idea that food should be simple, I offer my piece of nutritional advice: stock your fridge with whole foods, and avoid bags and boxes as much as possible. Don't be afraid to have fun with food. I know you're not from a family of foodies or even people who like to cook, but it's something that is worth learning.

As you watch people, especially athletes, work through their own relationship with food, don't get caught up in the comparison game. You'll hear story after story of athletes using food to leverage their performance. Lighter means faster, they'll say. Remember, dealing with disordered eating or an eating disorder is not a prerequisite for being a good athlete. Just because you're not tinkering with food or struggling to manage your diet doesn't mean you're not doing everything to be your best. Your body will naturally change, but don't think that means you need to fight it. It may take time to adapt to your new body, but likewise your body will adapt to new levels of training. It's silly to think you can outsmart or shortcut the process, and if you let it happen in its own time, you'll eventually end up with a build that is optimal for performance, appropriately lean and strong.

Paralysis by analysis is real in competition, and I think it can hold true here as well. It's easy to go down the wormhole of optimal nutrition, supplements, calorie counting, and so on. I think you've done a great job of not overthinking it thus far. Keep it simple, and keep it up.

STOPPING THE SWIRL
AND SEEKING BODY POSITIVITY

Identifying a purported ideal composition range includes moderately complex math and a need for lab-based testing. Transforming today's results by fueling yourself toward what *you* determine to be optimal is even more complex. But perhaps more difficult still is accepting and owning that there is no perfect weight or composition. Athletes and experts alike often struggle with this concept. After all, what we see in the media and on the racecourse or in the locker room often leads us to believe that thinner equals better equals faster. You know that there's much more to performance than one simple metric, but disputes over these measurements are common, and emotions often surround them. And once the stats are in, rarely are the conversations that follow helpful or motivational. American long-distance runner Kara Goucher reflects that along the road to medals and personal records, she suffered through years of criticism of her body and mandates to lose weight, all based on the assumption that manipulating the number on the scale would equal achievement. Today she knows that there's a better way. "I wish that instead of being taught about calories and numbers I had been taught about what kind of nutrition my body needed. I wish I had been told how important protein and hydration are after a hard session. How crucial it is to fuel with simple carbs before a long, hard sustained effort. Instead of counting calories, I wish earlier in my career I had used that mental energy to make sure I was getting the proper nutrients my body needed. I wish I had known how you can prep your body for a hard workout or help it recover faster just by fueling it properly. I think it would have prevented some unnecessary injuries and fatigue."

In other words, "Calorie counting be damned! Proper fueling eliminates the need to worry about calorie counting," says Goucher. Counting calories, ritualistically weighing yourself, and fretting over how you look in the mirror all carry a high risk of becoming unhealthy obsessions, capable of stealing from you your self-confidence and your love of sport. The negative swirl surrounding weight and body image is strong enough to drown male and female athletes alike.

Recently, men have been subjected to unfair criticism concerning how they look, especially when they deviate from the "ideal" weight and body composition. Still, women have always had it worse. Women have been put on display and subjected to idiotic standards of beauty or aesthetics for centuries. Even in modern times, such ridiculousness continues. Modern male European sand handball players wear tanks and long shorts, while females wear a uniform of close-fitting tops and bikini bottoms and are fined when they wear shorts instead. Female gymnasts and dancers compete in relatively revealing leotards and tights, while men wear formfitting shirts and pants.

Pervasive beliefs and sardonic comments about an athlete's "look" further hamper the efforts to change the conversation and move forward. Arrive at the starting line with additional muscle mass built to purposefully power across the pitch or along the racecourse, and cynics are quick to jump to conclusions about your likelihood to succeed.

Criticism of a person's body, whether said in an offhand manner, employed as a motivational technique, or even used to fill airtime, cuts deep, leaving wounds that linger for decades. On this topic, Kara Goucher reflects: "Every coach I have ever had has asked me at some point to eat less and lose weight, and over years, it messes with your mind. From comments of 'Here is where you hide your fat' to 'You can't afford to have a butt that big,' it's hard! All bodies are different, especially elite runner bodies. It is impossible for them to be the same. My body was a bit 'too tall' and 'too thick,' but I think that's why I could kick, why my career lasted so long, and why I could withstand such heavy training."

Women are far more likely than men to be criticized for the way they look, and unfortunately, women generally start with a lower level of self-confidence than men. This ongoing criticism along with unrealistic portrayals of bodies in the mass media have led to an

> **Pro Tip:** When in doubt, or when questioning if you look the part or are built to take on the task at hand, remember the wisdom of Kara Goucher: "Your body is a gift. It allows you to do what you love. Instead of trying to change it, appreciate it. And if you fuel it properly, it will become its own perfect shape."

unrelenting pursuit of some "ideal" yet unattainable physique. These factors play a role in the emergence of a pervasive dissatisfaction with one's body and heighten the risk of eating disorders. Most unfortunately, women are seemingly more in tune with such negative swirl, while men are often better equipped to ignore the noise. Recently, though, men too have begun to exhibit more dissatisfaction with their bodies, desiring to attain the current Western ideal of an unrealistically lean, muscular, V-shaped male body. Thus men, like women, are presented with an ideal physique that is difficult to achieve.

When does this negative swirl start? Sadly, disenchantment with one's body begins as early as elementary school, and self-disapproval reported by young girls quickly surpasses that of boys. Girls are more self-conscious about how their body weight affects their appearance and the majority are significantly concerned about their weight. *Overweight* girls feel even less body esteem, a decline that begins to affect boys once they are clinically *obese*. Upon reaching adolescence, boys are about equally divided between wanting to *lose* weight and wanting to add weight. (Grown men, on the other hand, tend to express a stronger desire to *lose* weight.) Body dissatisfaction in girls steadily increases from childhood to young womanhood, but even girls and women with the *lowest* levels of body dissatisfaction are still more displeased with their bodies than the males of the same age with the *highest* levels of dissatisfaction.

We must buck this trend right now by having powerfully positive conversations with girls (and boys) early and often. Intervention can change the reality that effectively overweight men consider themselves lighter than their actual weight while average-weight and underweight women still see themselves as heavier than they really are. Standing together to increase girls' self-confidence and body esteem is critical. Prevention of eating disorders and disordered eating stems from education and advocacy for change:

starting conversations to drive body positivity; advocating health and well-being and de-emphasizing body weight; and supporting mental health needs. It also involves modifications in approaches to sports: changing unhealthy sport rules and positioning a better relationship with food and self as "health and safety issues" rather than as "coaching issues."

Change begins with placing value on function over form. Young females are more likely to be dissatisfied with all factors—aesthetics, form, function, and all-around capabilities—so be the coach, mentor, parent, or friend who offers proper training to help growing athletes adapt to natural changes in physiology. Otherwise, girls may continue to drop out of sports at 1.5 times the rate of boys, and by age seventeen, more than half of females will have quit playing sports altogether. While people drop out of sports for many reasons, not all tied to body image, walking away from sports is walking away from developing the critical skills that tend to accompany participation in sports—teamwork, goal-setting, leadership training, and confidence-building.

DEAR YOUNGER, HUNGRY ME: KARA GOUCHER

Never content to sit and watch the world go by, Kara Goucher has embraced a life of reinvention and self-discovery. A professional runner with countless medals and achievements, she's evolved from Olympian to trail runner and sports commentator. She is a role-model mom to son Colt and wife to Adam, and she serves as a vocal advocate for women's sport, clean sport, and pushing the boundaries of what's possible. She has bravely stood up to running goliaths, suffering criticism, harassment, and even financial repercussions because of her unwillingness to remain silent. She has questioned coaching practices, experienced body criticism, and wrestled with her own self-doubt, but she has never relented in her quest to improve the future of sport. Her letter to her younger self will leave you inspired and wanting better for both yourself and our sport.

Dear Younger, Hungry Kara,

I wish you had all the wisdom and self-assuredness that I have now. I wish you could see that one meal will not determine the number on the scale or the results of a race. I wish you had the ability to see the future and see that when you stop starving your body and start nourishing it, the breakthroughs that you will have will be far greater than you ever hoped for.

When I was younger, I was taught what a calorie was. That a lot of calories add up to a pound. That pounds added to my body made me heavier. And that being heavier would slow me down.

This is all a myth, and you will eventually learn that. You will learn that by eating simple and pure carbs the night before a hard workout, you set yourself up for a great session the next day, with energy stores in your body. You will learn that by eating protein and calories after a run, you will recover faster and won't feel tired and wrecked after a workout. You will learn that if you treat your body with love and care, it will stay healthy, build muscle, and run faster than you ever imagined you could.

Someday you will go through puberty and it will be hard. You will get taller, gain weight, and you will even hear people talking about how your body has changed, slowed, gotten bigger. But this is what your body is supposed to be doing. It is changing and evolving. Eventually, you will be left with a new body. A body that can run more miles, lift more weights, and be stronger and more capable than your old body could ever be. Don't fight these changes. You are not failing by getting bigger, you are growing into your new self. Your stronger and more capable self. This self is the one that can achieve the biggest of dreams, things your old self could never do.

There will be parts of your body that you think aren't perfect. But let me tell you a fact that often feels like a secret: everyone's body is different. There is no perfect body, one way to be. The truth is that your body is perfect for YOU. You have the body you were meant to have. It is special in so many ways. Embrace who you are. It has gifts that are unique and perfect for you. It will take you wherever you want to go.

So do me a favor: treat your body well now. Love it, nourish it, treat it with care. It will support you, move you, help to achieve all you dream of and more. It will always be there for you, on good days and bad. Let it know that you appreciate it now. The sooner you fall in love with it, the sooner you will see all the amazing gifts and adventures you have right at your finger-tips!

Love,
Kara

AN INTRODUCTION TO ENERGY AND THE NUTRIENTS THAT MOVE US

CALORIES

Exercise and life itself require work. While you might see this work as fueled by grit and determination, the actual gas in the tank is the simple calorie. These units of energy are essential, although they are often vilified as the cause of weight gain.

Sometimes we do consume more calories than we need to support life, activity, and weight maintenance. And we can certainly make better choices about the foods we eat. For athletes, determining the number of calories to consume and from what sources can make the difference between achieving and being sidelined.

Calories come from carbohydrates, proteins, fats, and alcohol. In order to perform, we must have a readily available supply of these calories, and the source of these calories matters. Each nutrient plays a distinct important role in supporting health and performance; in fact the body has a remarkable ability to determine what kind(s) of fuel it needs for different types of workouts. When it's time to hit the accelerator, your body will rely on glucose. Going long? The body will draw from its glycogen and fat stores. Underfueled? The body will find the energy it needs by breaking down fat but also protein from the muscles. Clever and amazing as the body is, your job is to ensure that it has the right fuel at the right time. And it's not just fuel for exercise that matters, it's calories to support your day-to-day activities and your health and wellness. Let's spend some time talking about energy sources so you better understand what helps you move, what helps you thrive, and why it's essential to fuel the fire.

MACRONUTRIENTS (CARBOHYDRATES, PROTEIN, FATS)

You've got your energy needs mapped out, but where should those calories come from? Welcome to the world of macronutrients. Read on to determine the why, when, how, and sources of each nutrient.

Why Carbohydrates Matter

Carbohydrates are often painted as the bad guy, but for athletes, this makes little sense. Stored as glycogen and easily accessed glucose, carbs are the easiest form of calories for your body to convert to energy. They're also fairly easy to carry (ever tried to take a chicken breast or a stick of butter on the go?), widely available, and inexpensive. Admittedly, they are rarely as satiating as protein or as nourishing as fat. It's also easy to overdo your intake of carbs; snack foods tend to be packed with this nutrient in one of its simplest forms—sugar. But before you swear off carbs, understand that they are essential to performance and health, and your choice of sources matters.

Embrace carbs, for they provide critical fuel for the brain and central nervous system and can be put to work at various intensities and durations. Especially when you're pushing your limits and working at an incredibly high intensity, carbs easily outperform fat; they provide a greater yield of adenosine triphosphate (ATP) per volume of oxygen that can be delivered to the mitochondria. Basically, this means having carbs on board improves exercise efficiency (work rate/energy expenditure). Carbs empower overall exercise efficiency or the ability to translate chemical energy into movement. Carbs are broken down into glucose and stored in your muscles and liver in the form of glycogen. These stores change daily based on your intake and exercise. Stores are limited, and as levels are depleted, your body starts breaking down fat and protein for energy—which isn't optimal. As the intensity of your workout increases, so does the rate at which you burn through fuel. So you need to consume carbohydrate on a daily basis to prevent hitting E (and feeling miserable).

Some athletes train "low," without adequate carbohydrate. This practice typically fails to significantly improve performance, and the majority of available research suggests training with limited carbohydrate impairs intensity and duration, hampering your ability to go faster and longer.

Yes, you can reduce carb intake during the off-season, while recovering from an injury, or potentially on rest days, but anytime you have an intense or long workout on your schedule, you've got to fill up on carbs. At workout intensities near VO_2 max levels (that is to say, workout intensities ranging from those so intense you can't hold a conversation to those where breathing is labored but you can still manage small talk), most folks have enough glycogen on board to crank through a workout of thirty minutes to two hours. But this is true only if you are consistently consuming adequate carbs on a daily basis. In the book *Roar*, exercise physiologist Stacy Sims notes that "glycogen availability is the single biggest limiting factor for going strong and maintaining your effort and intensity for any type of prolonged exercise." Fail to top off the carb tank and you're basically setting yourself up to run into that dreaded wall hard and fast.

So why is it that carbohydrates get such a bad rap, being blamed for rising obesity rates in the United States and around the world? Carbohydrates themselves are not driving soaring obesity rates, but the types and volume of carbs most people choose. The makeup of your plate matters whether you're working to develop a lean body or trying to perform at your best in the classroom, on the field, or in the game of life. But in the standard American diet (yes, the acronym SAD is both fitting and ironic), approximately 42 percent of total calories comes from *low-quality* carbohydrate sources—thereby fueling the notion that carbs are to blame for poor health around the globe.

Classifying Carbs

When you consistently choose the highest-quality carbs—that is to say, those containing the most nutrients with the fewest unhealthy additives—you won't run into trouble. But how do you figure out which foods are "good" versus those which are "bad"? Instead of labeling foods good or bad, consider a food's purpose. Ask yourself, *How is this choice fueling my goals?* This approach will help you choose fewer lower-quality, nutrient-poor *sometimes foods* and prioritize *always foods* that supply health benefits rather than just a pick-me-up.

> **Pro Tip:** Some argue that carbs basically come in two varieties: quality carbs and substandard carbs. However, my go-to terms, sometimes foods and always foods, provide a more practical framework for most people. If you prefer, you could also view choices as good, better, and best. And if none of these labels work for you, simply view food as what it is—an apple, bread, a carrot, and so on.

ALWAYS CARBS. Fruits, vegetables, dairy, and whole grains are the best choices, the *always foods*. These high-quality carbs offer a plethora of nutrients you need, without the junk you don't. They supply fiber, antioxidants, phytonutrients, and essential vitamins and minerals. These choices need to be staples in your diet, no matter what your health, performance, or weight goals may be.

SOMETIMES CARBS. These foods offer little benefit beyond a quick hit of energy and an enticing taste. They're often easier to digest, so they can come in handy when you need a quick burst of energy or otherwise neglected to prime your tank with a meal hours earlier. For ideas, check out pre-workout fuel suggestions on page 183. Don't go overboard; fueling up day in and day out with cookies, crackers, refined grains, sweets, and empty-calorie snacks will leave you feeling like crap.

Remember, there's a huge difference between the carbs that come from refined grains in products such as white bread, bakery treats, and doughnuts and the carbs that come from whole grains like whole wheat pasta, oatmeal, buckwheat, quinoa, and farro, which have real health benefits. When you next sit down to a pre-run dinner or choose dining hall fare, reach for the highest-quality carbs available and find the fuel that supports your energy and your health.

Build a Better Plate: Carbs

What should these choices look like? Without fail, start with whole grain, fruits, and vegetables. No matter your goals, your mindset, your diet du jour, you should fill your plate with these superfoods *every single day*. Minimally processed ancient grains and garden gems offer varying amounts of calories—primarily from carbohydrates—along with fiber, antioxidants, phytochemicals, and nutrients to support your activity and your health. Occasionally, you might read an article or headline alleging one of the aforementioned is unhealthy or packed with sugar. *Wrong*. Ignore the hype. These foods are the foundation of good health, and I've yet to meet one person who has failed to reach their health, performance, or weight goals because their diet contained too many fresh fruits and vegetables.

Currently, just one in ten U.S. adults meets the federal fruit and vegetable recommendations (1½ to 2 cups of fruit per day and 2 to 3 cups of vegetables per day). In general, 1 serving of vegetables provides 5 grams of carbs and amounts to 1 cup of raw or ½ cup cooked, or 2 cups of raw, leafy greens. A serving of fruit typically contains 15 to 30 grams of carbs, depending on the sweetness and size of the fruit. A single serving is equal to 1 cup of chopped or sliced fresh fruit, 8 ounces of 100 percent fruit juice, ½ cup of dried fruit, or one medium-size piece of whole fruit. Whether fresh, frozen, or canned, just about all produce is an always carb!

Added benefit? By boosting your fruit and veggie intake, you'll also boost your fiber intake, which is critical to heart health. You can also find fiber in beans, nuts, seeds, and whole grains. Ideally, you should be eating at least 14 grams of fiber for every 1,000 calories you consume. For most of us, that equates to a goal of 25 to 30 grams of fiber per day. The vast majority (around 90 percent) of Americans do not come close to hitting this target; in fact, average daily fiber intake hovers around a measly 17 grams or less. Higher fiber intake is linked to lower body weight, so by simply meeting the goal of 30 grams a day, you can hit those lean body goals while simultaneously fueling health and performance goals.

Eat Those Veggies, Please

Many people maintain that they don't consume more fresh fruits and vegetables because fresh fruits and vegetables cost too much or are inconvenient to prepare. Other people say that they don't know how to prepare these foods or that they simply don't like the taste and texture of them. Here are some solutions for all the above:

PREP FOR PLANTS: Map out your snacks and meals for the week, making sure each incorporates a wide array of fruits and vegetables in various forms—fresh, frozen, canned, dried, pureed in a smoothie. Dried fruits and smoothies are great options before workouts. Post-workout, build your meal with fruits and vegetables first, and combine these with other nutrient-dense foods like whole grains, low-fat dairy, and lean protein.

PLAN AHEAD: Fill your cart with fresh veggies for dinner tonight and frozen or canned ones for the days ahead. Shop sales. Shop seasonally. Stock up as you're able. Keep smoothie starters and dried fruits on hand for easy snacks and recipes.

PLANTS ON REPEAT: Make it a habit to consistently choose plant foods, and soon adding fruits and vegetables to meals and snacks will become automatic. It's as simple as adding berries or a banana to a morning smoothie, enjoying some baba ghanoush with a handful of broccoli and sliced bell pepper as a midmorning snack, and starting dinner with a veggie-filled salad. Explore new forms and flavors until you find a variety of go-tos.

Adding More *Always* Foods

You likely have a pretty good idea about which foods to choose always and which ones should fill your plate only sometimes. Follow these simple steps to always (See what I did there?) find wholesome choices:

1. **Shop wisely.** On grocery store shelves, if the food doesn't have a label, this is assurance you're choosing wisely. Most non-packaged goods like fruits, vegetables, and bulk grains don't typically come with a nutrition facts panel. If the food has a label and an ingredient panel, favor foods with a short list of ingredients. Look for words like *whole grain* instead of *enriched,* which means the grain has been processed and stripped of naturally occurring nutrients.

2. **Choose simply prepared.** In the dining hall and at restaurants, choose simply prepared grains and veggies—steamed, boiled, grilled, lightly sautéed—rather than breaded, fried, and sauced selections.

3. **Skip sugar-riddled snacks and sides.** Most of us should be consuming no more than 25 grams of added sugar a day. You'll know a packaged food is rich in added sugars when one of the first two ingredients—which are listed in order by weight—is sugar or some other form of this caloric sweetener.

4. **Shop the perimeter of the store.** The interior of any grocery store typically contains foods with lots of additives to ensure a long shelf life. Perishable fresh foods are most often stored in coolers and display cases on the perimeter of the store. Venture to the center of the store for raw bulk staples like whole grains, canned beans, dry cereals, and the few other items you simply can't live without.

5. **Give yourself a break.** Sometimes you're just at the mercy of convenience. Sometimes sugar or white bread is all you have to work with. Other times you have

access to any food imaginable. When you choose a food, simply ask yourself, *Is this the best choice for me?*

Carbohydrates: How Much Is Enough?

How many carbs do you need to fuel your day? Many athletes skip the math, instead consuming servings throughout the day and timing these servings so they have fuel in the tank when they need to hit go.

If you're starting from scratch and want to map out your day with precision, here are three commonly used methods that I've seen work:

1. **START SIMPLE.** Consider what percentage of your total calories should come from carbs. In general, athletes in strength and team sports should aim for an intake of about 40 percent of calories from carbs, and athletes in long-distance and endurance sports should aim for an intake closer to 65 percent. Once you determine your starting point (remember, it's acceptable—in fact it's a good practice—to let your intake evolve over time until you find a blend that works for you), look down at your plate. If 65 percent of your calories comes from carbs, about 65 percent of the plate should be filled with a mix of whole grains, fruit, and so on. If 40 percent of the plate should be filled with carbs, then aim for smaller portions of the same sources and round out the remainder with lean protein and fat.

2. **CONSIDER TOTAL GRAMS NEEDED.** Using the same percentages outlined above, estimate the number of calories you need and multiply by 40 to 65 percent, depending on the demands of your sport and lifestyle. Divide this number by 4 (there are 4 calories per gram of carb), and you'll arrive at the number of grams you need to consume. As you track your intake throughout the day, you can record the number of carbs (and protein and fats) you consume and tweak your intake until you find your perfect plate.

3. **DO THE MATH.** Multiply your body weight by the recommended number of grams per pound. Rounded ranges are based on clinical data from performance-oriented trials, and the number of grams per pound naturally fluctuates based on demands of training and intensity. I've worked with athletes who require more carbs than the recommendations below to fuel their intense training, and I've worked with athletes who require slightly fewer carbs to perform at their best. You'll need to experiment until you arrive at a plan perfect for you.

Goal-Driven Carb Calculations

GOAL: Off-season body composition goals or rehabbing an injury.

PRO TIP: Favor satiating, recovery-oriented protein over carbohydrates. Time your carb intake (see "The Right Fuel at the Right Time" on page 176) to promote high carb availability pre-workout, mid-workout, and during the recovery restocking phase.

NEEDS: Aim for 1.3 to 2.3 grams per pound of body weight (again, don't skimp on protein).

GOAL: Fuel your baseline workouts (about 1 hour per day) and your day.

PRO TIP: Choose *always* carbs throughout the day and round out your plate with purposeful protein and fat.

NEEDS: Aim for 2.3 to 3.2 grams of carb per pound of body weight. For best results, time this intake around your workouts.

GOAL: Fuel your moderate- to high-intensity race training, in-season practices, and workouts that last 1 to 3 hours a day.

PRO TIP: Choose nutrient-rich, carbohydrate-rich foods across your day and at each meal.

NEEDS: Aim for 2.5 to 4.5 grams of carb per pound of body weight. Hit the high end of this range on intense training days.

GOAL: Survive and thrive during Ironman training, marathon hell-week training, or a series of back-to-back two-a-days.

PRO TIP: Prioritize carbs and protein over fat and consume carbs pre-workout, mid-workout, and post-workout.

NEEDS: Aim for 3.5 to 5.5 grams of carb per pound of body weight. Hit the high end of this range on intense training days.

Remember, these guidelines are meant to be a starting point. Adapt these recommended ranges to best meet your personal needs. If you find yourself getting prematurely tired during workouts, up your intake slightly. If you feel energized but are not making any progress toward a weight goal, take it down a notch, and so on.

Take-Home Points

▸ The vast majority of us want and need carbs. Higher levels of activity demand more of this efficient fuel source. Plan your plate accordingly.

▸ Some sources are better than others. Consider *sometimes* carbs and *always* carbs and let your health, wellness, and performance goals determine the amount and type of carbs consumed and the timing of the intake. Even if you're working toward healthy weight loss, you still need carbs to avoid feeling fatigued and burning protein for energy.

▸ When looking to hit a performance goal, you'll need a steady intake of carbs throughout the day to keep your glycogen levels high and your body ready to hit go whenever the opportunity for a sweat session might arise.

▸ When you are chasing a return to performance or trying to hit lean body goals, carb intake is still essential, and timing matters. Choose fewer *sometimes* carbs but keep the *always* sources that provide nutrient density. Time these choices so you have enough energy in the tank to crank through a workout and still find the mental release, metabolic adaptations, and performance gains you're seeking.

Why Proteins Matter

If your daily intake of fuel is similar to that of athletes whose typical food records I've re-viewed over the years, there's a solid chance you're not getting enough protein. As Olympian and half-marathon American record holder Ryan Hall has said, "I wish I would have eaten more protein. I bought into the whole 'your body can only absorb twenty grams of protein in one sitting' line and wasn't recovering optimally. I was craving big pieces of salmon like crazy, but I wouldn't allow myself to take in more than four ounces in one sitting." Hall started working with a nutritionist, who discovered that he was deficient in protein. Hall happily upped his intake to include three 12-ounce steaks per week for nearly a month until his blood protein levels improved. The outcome? A few months later, Hall ran his best marathon ever.

Whether you're an Olympic-caliber athlete, an aspiring elite, or a fitness enthusiast, never underestimate the power of protein. And make sure that your intake includes varied high-quality sources paced evenly throughout your day.

Built on a foundation of amino acids, proteins are responsible for a plethora of metabolic reactions and are essential in maintaining a well-functioning immune system, bone and tendon integrity, strong muscles, healthy skin, hair, and nails, and the list goes on. Adaptations to training rely on an adequate intake of protein to supply essential amino acids, especially the amino acid leucine, which jump-starts the synthesis of muscle protein.

There's also a clear link between protein intake and body composition, stemming from increased satiety and thermogenesis and the capacity to preserve metabolically active muscle tissue. (Lean mass is protected during times of weight loss, while fat is shed, to a degree.) Protein *does* help fend off hunger and it *does* take more energy for the body to digest, but it is *not* a magic bullet for weight loss, despite the headlines and claims you might encounter. But a greater intake of protein is critical if you consistently fail to adequately fuel up on carbs or if you don't take in enough calories. This is because your body is likely to use some protein for energy, in addition to fulfilling the host of other functions protein does throughout the day.

Even when the body is properly fueled, an adequate supply of protein is essential during times of intense training. Workouts lead to exercise-induced muscle breakdown, and muscles must be rebuilt. Also, small amounts of protein are used for energy, and additional protein beyond the bare minimum RDA is needed to support gains in lean muscle mass. This is why so many nutrition experts denounce the headlines that claim people eat too much protein. Current thinking is that serious athletes need far more protein in their daily diet than what is recommended, just to support the activities of daily living. Instead, the focus has pivoted to providing enough protein at optimal times to halt breakdown and begin the rebuilding process.

Spoiler alert: You're probably not eating enough protein. Many people think that we all consume far too much protein, but this is not true. Most individuals eat sufficient protein for health but not for performance, training adaptations, or adaptation to menstrual cycle phases. When athletes do consume enough protein, it's generally because they are eating enough to meet the demands of their sport, and their overall energy intake provides enough protein. In athletes who are cutting calories, those who eat a limited variety of foods, or those who are focused on carbs to fuel intensity, protein intake can fall short.

Protein: How Much Is Enough?

▸ The Recommended Dietary Allowance (RDA) established the baseline protein needs for the general population. It's possibly enough to support health and the activities of daily living, but it is ***definitely inadequate to support performance***.

▸ The RDA for adults is 0.36 g/lb/day (0.8 g/kg/day).

▸ Additional guidance is provided by the Daily Value (DV), a reference amount listed on a packaged food's nutrition facts panel and which provides insight into whether a food is rich in a nutrient in the context of daily diet. The DV for protein is 50 g/day.

Exercise demands support from protein, and research suggests athletes require at least two times the RDA. Needs are higher for athletes who are undergoing intense training, for athletes nearing or into Masters age category competition, and for most women, especially during the high hormone phase. Higher protein recommendations serve to augment rapid protein turnover in tissues during repair and remodeling and metabolic adaptations initiated by training.

- ► Active individuals need to aim for an intake between 0.55 and 1.0 g/lb/day (1.2–2.0 g/kg/day), spread evenly over the day.

- ► Higher intakes (beyond 1.0 g/lb) may be indicated for short training blocks that demand intensified training or when reducing overall energy intake.

Your personal requirements are fluid, based on some of the following factors:

- ► "Trained" status or not: experienced athletes may require less.

- ► Phase and demands of training: new and challenging, or high-intensity and/or high-frequency sessions push protein needs toward the high end of the range.

- ► Overall carbohydrate availability: low availability increases the body's demand for protein.

- ► Age: older athletes are less efficient at absorption and utilization of protein.

- ► Total energy needs plus availability: more total calories means more calories from protein. In addition, adequate energy from other sources spares amino acids for protein synthesis.

- ► Phase of the menstrual cycle: as you'll learn in "The Impact of Menstruation" (see page 211), needs fluctuate throughout your cycle.

Is it possible to consume too much of a good thing? We've all seen plates piled high with chicken breast topped with steak, but there's rarely a downside to occasionally consuming an amount of protein that surpasses your actual needs. The tolerable upper limit for protein is about 1.6 g/lb/day (3.5 g/kg/day). Chronically excessive intake may have negative implications for bone, digestive, renal, and vascular health. Rare is the endurance athlete, or female athlete, who habitually consumes protein levels near or exceeding this tolerable upper limit. But if your daily intake consists of protein smoothies at every snack and multiple chicken breasts at every meal, it may be time to cut back.

Build a Better Plate: Protein

Packed with adequate levels of essential amino acids, high-quality dietary proteins help support general health as well as performance-centric lean muscle maintenance, repair, and synthesis. But with so much to choose from and an abundance of purported benefits to consider, it can be near impossible to sift through the noise and find a quality protein. So let's start at the building blocks of protein: amino acids.

> **Pro Tip:** When it comes to protein, quality is not the same as quantity, and one gram of protein is not necessarily the same as another. Start with the source; amino acid content matters. Follow the lead of Joan Benoit Samuelson and eat local, high-quality protein, and a variety of it. And as you grow older, be sure to add more protein to your plate; as we age, our bodies become less efficient at synthesizing protein and muscle breakdown accelerates.

Your body breaks down protein into individual amino acids. There are twenty different amino acids—nine essential ones, which you need to source from food, and eleven nonessential ones, which your body can build from other amino acids. These building blocks are pooled in the body and reassembled to create new proteins and perform various biological functions. Different sources of protein contain different combinations and concentrations of amino acids, and the amounts and types of these help determine if a protein is of high quality.

Classifying Protein

When determining what makes a high-quality source of protein, experts consider amino acid content and digestibility (highly digestible proteins contain amino acids readily available to the body), and the resulting availability of amino acids to support metabolic function.

Simplify your choices by giving preference to sources high in the essential amino acids (branched-chain amino acids valine, leucine, and isoleucine; lysine, threonine, tryptophan, methionine, phenylalanine, and histidine). Food labels rarely indicate protein quality, but you can be confident that animal sources (save a few mentioned below) are high in all the essential amino acids, making them complete choices.

While plant proteins offer health benefits beyond amino acid content, these choices are naturally low in select essential amino acids and thus incomplete. Additionally, plant proteins are more difficult to digest, so their bioavailability is also compromised.

A Protein Deep Dive: Animal and Vegetable Sources

ANIMAL PROTEINS

Animal proteins range from nutrient-dense beef, pork, chicken, eggs, and fish to drinkable dairy, bone broths, and shakes (whey and casein protein powders). Top choices continue to fly off the shelves; meat jerky alone is a $1.4 billion market, and per capita intake of red meat plus poultry is forecast to hit 223 pounds in 2022, one of the highest levels recorded since 1960.

Most all animal sources, except collagen and related bone broths, are sources of high-quality protein that can act as your sole source of protein if need be. Collagen protein, while popular and used for various reasons like joint health, is high in three nonessential amino acids—glycine, proline, and hydroxyproline—making this an inadequate protein to support total body health and performance.

Dairy protein should be a mainstay in your diet (unless you find yourself allergic to or intolerant of milk or are vegan), as it's high in leucine, an amino acid responsible for initiating muscle protein synthesis. Dairy is generally convenient, relatively inexpensive, and has been extensively studied. The benefits of dairy hinge on the presence of casein and whey—two ingredients naturally present in milk. Casein, a slow-digesting protein, provides a steady stream of amino acids to muscles over many hours, while whey is known to be rapidly digested and therefore quickly repairs, restores, and rebuilds muscles after a workout.

PLANT PROTEINS

Plant proteins are growing (no pun intended) in popularity, convenience, taste, and availability. This is due largely in part to consumers seeking out more protein from a greater variety of sources. Plant protein remains incomplete and less anabolic than animal-based protein, but if you consume a variety of different kinds of plant protein, you are likely to receive health and performance benefits from them.

Athletes who rely on plant protein should be careful to combine sources or even add some animal protein in order to be better equipped to rebuild and make strength gains. Soy may be the exception here—its amino acid profile is nearly complete, but it lacks adequate leucine (unless you're willing to consume an awful lot of tofu and edamame) to jumpstart muscle protein synthesis.

Vegans can meet their protein needs by effectively eating more, but if your sources of plant protein are neither varied nor used throughout the day to complement each other, you're just spinning your wheels. No matter how much of one specific source of plant protein you consume, there's a good chance that you'll be missing essential amino acids.

Protein recommendations and intake vary across a spectrum. The amount needed is dependent on your personal requirements plus the overall quality of the protein of your diet. If you consume only plant-based protein, you'll need to eat more and might consider supplementing with branched-chain amino acid supplements to compensate for the lower quality of the protein and to ensure an adequate intake of essential amino acids. So if you are going plant-based, remember, you need to choose purposefully, but the effort will be worthwhile; longevity studies suggest that diets including higher intakes of plant-based protein and fat and less animal-based protein and fat often lead to better health outcomes.

Pro Tips to Get More Protein on Your Plate

1. When you dine, make sure your plate includes a source of protein. Include at least 15 grams of protein at snacks and at least 30 grams at meals, depending on your overall pursuits.

2. Going back for seconds? Skip empty calories and simple starches and instead have a small chicken breast, a scoop of lentils, or another lean protein choice.

3. Plan carefully and keep an open mind. If plant protein is your jam, you need variation across your day. Switch up your choices to ensure you're getting a variety of amino acids as well as a variety of micronutrients.

4. Don't struggle—grab a smoothie. When it comes to taste, texture, availability, and protein sourcing options, protein powders are now mainstream and can even be delicious. Check in with your team dietitian for a safe and reputable choice. (Brands carrying an NSF Certified for Sport or an Informed Choice seal of approval are typically recommended for athletes.) Avoid any brand with "proprietary blends" and supplements added. Choose one with 20 to 30 grams of protein per serving, and limit added sugars and fat.

5. Keep it simple. If you're seeking optimal protein intake without the worry of balancing amino acid intake and quality, your best bet is to consume a variety of proteins from animal and plant sources throughout the day.

What Counts as a Serving?

Refer to the table below when planning your day, keeping in mind the contribution of different foods. Space your intake of protein evenly across the day and include at least one serving of protein per meal.

Note: Data is provided by the USDA's FoodData Central, and all values are for cooked or canned items unless otherwise indicated.

Protein Choice	Serving Size	Protein Content (g)
LEAN MEAT	3–4 oz. steak (round, filet) 3 oz. ground beef sirloin, pork, bison 3 oz. pork tenderloin or loin roast	20–25 g
POULTRY	3 oz. chicken or turkey breast 3 oz. rotisserie chicken	25–30 g
SEAFOOD	3 oz. tuna, canned in water 3 oz. fresh fish (cod, salmon, trout) 3 oz. shrimp	17–23 g
EGGS	1 egg or 2 egg whites	6–7 g
NUTS AND SEEDS	1 oz. nuts (23 almonds, 49 pistachios, 14 walnut halves) 1 oz. seeds (85 pumpkin, 3.5 tbsp sunflower seeds, hulled, roasted) 2 tablespoons peanut butter or almond butter	4–7 g
BEANS AND PEAS	½ cup cooked beans (black, kidney, pinto, or white beans) ½ cup cooked peas (chickpeas, cowpeas, lentils, or split peas) ½ cup baked beans or refried beans ½ cup (4 oz.) tofu ¼ cup roasted soybeans 4 tablespoons hummus	7–8 g 7–8 g 6–7 g 18–21 g 17 g 4–5 g

Why Fats Matter

It wasn't that long ago that people viewed fats and oils as villainous. Energy-dense and providing 9 calories a gram, fats and oils (or *lipids,* as they're known in the technical literature) handily intimidated fitness enthusiasts, athletes, and really just about anyone cutting calories who perhaps justifiably believed fat was a major obstacle to getting svelte fast.

What was missed in this equation was the nutritional value and resounding health benefits that healthy fat choices bring to the table. We've reversed our former thinking, and now high-fat diets are über popular and one of the top diet trends. As a clinician, I've seen tremendous health benefits in following high-fat diets and I've also seen some miserable athletic performances when carbs and protein were neglected in favor of fat. As a nutrition expert who believes every food fits (admittedly, some better than others), I'm encouraged to see general opinion is undergoing a shift in perspective, as more of this essential nutrient is included in meal plans and menus and is jotted down on food records.

The Value of Fat

Nourishing fats should have a presence in your diet, whatever your specific health and performance goals may be. Dietary fat has many functions in the body, the primary role being to serve as an energy source while at rest and also during times of activity. Whether circulating throughout your plasma in the form of free fatty acids, existing in your muscle in the form of triglycerides, or providing energy once mobilized from adipose (fat) tissue, fat is a plentiful source of fuel. And as endurance training continues and metabolic adaptations occur, fat becomes even more readily available to fuel the muscle.

The utilization of this fuel source when your cells can't access other energy sources, such as glucose, is critical to survival. Fat provides essential fuel for the body during periods of dietary restriction or illness or in response to altered metabolism due to a variety of factors. A balanced plate inclusive of fat helps thwart blood glucose spikes and consequent insulin spikes, potentially preventing an increase in cortisol levels. Why does this matter? Chronically high blood glucose levels increase the risk of diabetes, and an increase in cortisol often leads to a buildup of abdominal fat. Fat also offers protection against internal temperature fluctuations, protects one's internal organs, and allows estrogen to function properly, therefore assuring a more regular menstrual cycle and the resultant preservation of fertility and bone health.

Both exogenous fat intake and endogenous fat stores facilitate absorption of essential

fat-soluble vitamins—the very vitamins that support your pursuit of health and high performance. Fat-soluble vitamin A is critical for vision as well as reproduction, cell differen-
tiation, and bone formation. The sunshine vitamin, vitamin D, which is actually a hormone,
is not prevalent in the food supply, so heightened absorption is critical to calcium status
and bone health as well as a host of other physiological processes. A powerful antioxidant,
vitamin E supports immune health and is commonly found in high-fat foods (and absorption is facilitated by such sources), and exercise may further increase your need for E. Finally, vitamin K should not be overlooked, as it's necessary for blood clotting and bone
health. Research has found that vitamin K supplementation and enhanced absorption are
even more important in athletes, since intense exercise can have a metabolic cost, weaken-
ing bones.

When it comes to nutrient density and overall nutritional value, the type and source of
fat make a huge difference. The fats you choose can move you toward or away from your
overall health goals. For example, while unsaturated fats can improve your cholesterol levels and thus your heart health, trans fats negatively impact heart health by altering your
total cholesterol ratio: raising overall total cholesterol and raising the levels of bad cholesterol (LDL) while decreasing the levels of healthy cholesterol (HDL). Ultimately, frequent
intake of this source of fat can increase your risk of developing heart disease.

The jury is still out on the full impact or benefit of saturated fats. These fats have been
shown to impact total cholesterol levels, but many large long-term studies have failed to
link intake of saturated fat to risk of heart disease. In fact, some research points to select
components of saturated fats, such as stearic acid, as being helpful in balancing cholesterol
levels or even in thwarting inflammation. The important finding of these potential benefits
is the source of the saturated fat. Natural and unprocessed sources, including dairy, grass-
fed beef, and eggs get a green light. Caution should be employed when consuming the saturated fats (as well as sugar, additives, and so forth) found in highly processed hot dogs, deli
meats, bakery items, and sweets.

In general, experts continue to recommend full elimination of trans fats. I typically
suggest a thoughtful restriction of saturated fat intake. If you're not sure where to start
when selecting the best source of fats and oils for your health and performance, look to
plants, not animals. Largely unsaturated fats from most plants, nuts, and seeds promote

optimal health. Conversely, the fats found in processed foods, lard, and untrimmed meats are highly saturated, and some longitudinal studies point to poorer outcomes with higher intakes of animal fats.

Fat: How Much Is Enough?

While many current and popular approaches to eating call for the vast majority of calories to come from fat, the AMDR (Acceptable Macronutrient Distribution Range) suggests that fat provide between 20 and 35 percent of your daily calories. Recent dietary intake data suggests that average American adults receive some 32 percent of their daily caloric intake from fat. For athletes, extreme fat intake, be it severely high or low, promotes neither optimal performance nor health. Yes, some fat-adapted athletes have found success on the ketogenic diet, and some athletes find their calorie goals easier to hit when modifying their fat intake. While research in this field continues, at this point, there is limited support for extremes; neither high-fat intake devoid of carbs nor low-fat plans devoid of adequate micronutrients and essential fatty acids point performance in the right direction. In fact, significant restriction of fat intake to less than 15 percent of daily energy not only fails to provide a performance benefit but may ultimately increase the athlete's risk of injury. Simply increasing the percentage of calories from fat may reduce the risk of future injury. Research involving seasoned female runners (20-plus miles per week) found that those who consumed a diet significantly lower in total fat and lower in percentage of total calories from fat (27 percent versus 30 percent) were more likely to be sidelined by injury compared to runners who consumed more total fat, or the recommended 30 percent of their daily energy from fat.

If you're actively working to reduce overall caloric intake and find that consuming fat in the hours pre-workout messes with your GI system, and/or if you're in the middle of upping carb intake to load glycogen, it's perfectly acceptable to occasionally decrease your fat intake. Consume less fat during the hours pre- and post-workout, since these fueling sessions should be focused on carbs, protein, and fluid. Remember, don't go long stretches of time with significantly reduced fat; failing to consume at least 20 percent of total calories from fat leads to reduced intake of key nutrients, including fat-soluble vitamins and essential fatty acids.

Classifying Fat: Sources to Fuel You

Sources of fat are typically classified based on their chemical structure, and this structure has an impact on health. In general, unsaturated fats are found in liquid form, as their weaker chemical structure includes any number of double bonds that are not completely saturated (with hydrogen atoms) and therefore can bend and move easily. Imagine these liquid oils as moving more easily through your arteries. Saturated fats have a robust makeup with no double bonds, so they are instead stiff. As is true with other macronutrients, for optimal health, sources matter. Here's a look at foods to choose.

UNSATURATED FAT

Unsaturated fats are able to benefit total cholesterol and LDL levels while guarding against heart disease. You'll find unsaturated fats in vegetable and nut oils, including almond, avocado, canola, olive, peanut, pecan, and pistachio. The umbrella term *unsaturated fat* includes both monounsaturated fatty acids (MUFAs) and polyunsaturated fatty acids (PUFAs), classifications based on the chemical structure of these lipids. Most sources contain a mix of MUFAs and PUFAs, and since both types offer health benefits, there's no need to lose sleep trying to determine exact intake of each.

Wondering why everyone says to eat more fish or supplement with omega-3s? Omega-3s are essential fatty acids (that is to say, you must obtain them from food), and these PUFAs protect against inflammation, help regulate cellular functions, and maintain brain, muscle, and nerve function. Eating more foods rich in these fatty acids, along with omega-6s, another essential nutrient, can lead to a reduced risk of heart disease and protect against chronic inflammatory diseases and age-related brain decline. It's not difficult to find sources of omega-6 oils, since many common oils like soy and canola are rich in this nutrient. You'll need to work a bit harder to add in sources of omega-3 oils; these are commonly found in fish oils and fatty cold-water fish, shellfish, walnuts, hempseed hearts, and flaxseed.

TRANS FAT

When it comes to overly processed trans fat, consume as little of this as possible. Intake of trans fats has been linked to poor blood lipid levels, an increased risk of cardiovascular disease and stroke, and other undesirable health outcomes. Trans fats are incredibly shelf stable, allowing the processed foods they are commonly found in to remain on your grocer's shelf longer without going rancid. Food manufacturers have worked diligently to eliminate many of the ingredients that contain trans fats. However, while many foods claim 0 grams of trans fats per serving, be aware that rounding comes into play. Foods with less than 0.5 grams per serving can still be labeled as trans fat free, so steer clear of foods containing partially hydrogenated oils. Higher levels of trans fat are typically found only in commercial baked goods, baking mixes, empty-calorie snack items, and junk foods that you're likely working to limit anyway.

MEDIUM-CHAIN FATTY ACIDS

Medium-chain triglycerides (MCTs) supply quick energy and, according to some fans, an increased metabolic burn accompanied by mental focus. MCTs are found in varying degrees in coconut oil, palm kernel oil, and butter, and also in powdered and liquid supplements. The chemical makeup of MCTs is a significantly smaller lipid in comparison with saturated and unsaturated fats of longer lengths. Potential benefits of a diet rich in MCT oil revolves around this smaller structure.

Due to their shorter chain length, MCTs can be quickly absorbed in the gastrointestinal tract and transported to the liver via the portal circulation without the extra steps typically required to digest a longer-chain source of fat. As a result, MCTs are quickly used for energy by the muscles, the surrounding tissues, and even the brain (typically while in a fasting or ketogenic state), rather than being stored for future use. Some research points to the potential of a diet rich in MCT oil to impede fat storage, increase thermogenesis (metabolic burn), and also increase satiety. The scientific findings are mixed, but published data suggest that including a daily dose of MCT oil may result in a negative energy balance and weight loss through increased energy expenditure and lipid oxidation. Frequent replacement of dietary fat with sources of MCT could potentially induce modest reductions in body weight and composition without adversely affecting your lipid profile. But adding the star ingredient in keto coffee to your diet poses a risk. Your gastrointestinal system must adapt to it, and most people experience GI distress when they first try this source of fat. I recommend starting slowly and on an off day until you know if it works for you.

SATURATED FAT

It's easy to spot saturated fats because they are typically solid at room temperature. Sources include animal-based butter, lard, bacon, marbled meat, poultry with the skin, and dairy products; plant-based sources are coconut oil, palm oil, and cocoa butter. Given the potential of saturated fat to negatively impact heart health, the most recent edition of the *Dietary Guidelines for Americans* recommends consuming less than 10 percent of daily calories from saturated fat. Some 70 to 75 percent of adults typically exceed this recommendation. This overconsumption is understandable, given that for every 1,000 calories you consume, your intake of saturated fat should be less than 11 grams, or the amount found in 1½ tablespoons of butter, 1 tablespoon of coconut oil, or ⅓ cup of heavy cream.

There's significant controversy over the long-held belief that saturated fats increase the risk of heart disease, perhaps illustrating that the jury is still out on exactly what makes up an optimal diet (if such a thing even exists). The American Heart Association maintains that decades of research still support lowering your risk of heart disease by replacing saturated fats with the heart-healthy fats in nuts, seeds, avocados, fish, and plant-based oils and fats—so moderation may be the key. Dr. Jenna Bell notes that "saturated fat notwithstanding, data indicates that increasing 'good fats' (like those found in nuts, seeds, avocados, fish, and plant oils) is good for your heart and health." She adds that in spite of some research supporting the nutritional value of coconut oil or high-fat dairy products, few studies have shown that saturated fatty acids, specifically, are essential in the diet.

While the scientists continue to debate, endorsing a diet high in saturated fat is unwarranted. "Instead of shopping for nutrients, shop for food. Vary your choices, try new things, bring diversity to dinner. Aim for an interesting approach to food—flavorful and healthful. You can have your meat and plant-based too!" The bottom line, according to Dr. Bell: "It's not about one nutrient—it's about our whole lifestyle."

Understanding Micronutrients and Supplements

Macronutrients serve to provide energy and effectively fuel you. Micronutrients—essential vitamins and minerals—are needed in minute quantities, support health, and can effectively make or break your performance. Micronutrients are best found in nutrient-dense foods, so you can assure a sufficient intake of them by consuming a variety of foods; prioritizing foods with natural color, such as fruits and vegetables; and including cereals, whole grains and fortified grains, lean protein, and dairy. Fortified foods, many sports nutrition products, and dietary supplements also contain a mix of additional micronutrients. Consuming these foods and supplements, while not always necessary, lends additional insurance that you're meeting your needs.

Defining Nutrient Density

The nutrient density of a food is the ratio of essential nutrients in the food to the energy content of the food for the amount generally consumed. There's a lot of debate concerning the exact components of nutrient density or the potential health benefits of foods, but for your health and performance, you can effectively consume a nutrient-dense diet by choosing more *always* foods, which tend to offer more nutritional bang for your calorie buck.

> **Pro Tip:** Sometimes you need energy-dense foods to fuel your workout and power your day. As American Olympic long-distance runner Molly Seidel puts it, "I'm tired of hearing about nutrient-dense foods. For a runner who is still unpacking and navigating an eating disorder, I'm focused on taking in adequate calories and eating mindfully. When I'm in heavy training and need three thousand to four thousand plus calories each day to fuel high mileage, I need energy-dense foods. I can't get enough calories from broccoli alone!" Seidel is right that there's a time and place for both energy-dense foods and nutrient-dense foods.

Heavy training demands energy-dense foods, but you can have the best of both worlds. Employ your own nutrient timing skills (see page 179) to top off your tank in the hours before training. During the hours you are focused on recovery and restocking, you have the freedom and time to choose nutrient-dense foods. In other words, when you can, choose more *always* foods and fewer *sometimes* foods.

Micronutrients: Why, When, How Much?

To help you bring the nutrients you need onto your plate, the table on the following page outlines a mix of micronutrient intake recommendations across the stages of life, explaining why these specific nutrients matter and where they come from, and what happens should you fall short. These recommendations are based on established Dietary Reference Intakes and also from expert sources such as the latest edition of the *Dietary Guidelines for Americans* and the American College of Obstetricians and Gynecologists, as well as practical advice from practitioners and clinical data.

> **Pro Tip:** *Dietary Reference Intakes (DRI) is the umbrella term for the set of reference values used to plan and assess the nutrient intakes of healthy people. These values vary by age and gender and include:*
>
> > ▸ **Recommended Dietary Allowance (RDA):** *the average daily level of intake sufficient to meet the nutrient requirements of nearly all (97–98 percent) healthy people.*
> >
> > ▸ **Adequate Intake (AI):** *just enough; established when evidence is insufficient to develop an RDA and set at a level assumed to ensure nutritional adequacy.*
> >
> > ▸ **Tolerable Upper Intake Level (UL):** *maximum daily intake unlikely to cause adverse health effects.*

MICRONUTRIENTS AND THE FOODS TO CHOOSE

Nutrient	What It Does (Function)	How Much Is Needed Each Day	Possible Effects of a Deficiency	Find It In
VITAMINS				
VITAMIN E (ALPHA-TOCOPHEROL)	Vitamin E acts as an antioxidant, fighting off the body's invaders through the immune system. It may prevent oxidative damage during exercise. Vitamin E also helps with healthy blood flow, keeping the muscles moving and the heart pumping.	15 mg 19 mg: lactation	Vitamin E deficiency can lead to feelings of muscle weakness and possibly a weakened immune system.	Wheat germ, almonds, sunflower seeds, spinach, broccoli, fortified cereals and juices, sunflower/safflower oil
VITAMIN A (RAE)	Vitamin A supports healthy vision and helps form healthy bones, teeth, and soft tissues. It supports a healthy immune system by supporting mucous membrane and skin integrity, the first line of defense.	700 mcg RAE 770 mcg RAE: pregnancy 1,300 mcg RAE: lactation	Vitamin A deficiency can result in blurry vision, which can impact performance in the classroom or on the field. Deficiency can also impact cell differentiation and reproductive health.	Dark leafy greens, broccoli, squash, carrots, cantaloupe, mangoes, salmon, sweet potatoes, pumpkin
VITAMIN D (CHOLECALCIFEROL)	Also known as the sunshine vitamin, vitamin D plays a critical role in helping your body absorb calcium, leading to strong bones and healthy muscles. This fat-soluble vitamin also supports the immune system and nervous system to function at their best.	15 mcg or 600 IU 1,000–2,000 IU D_3 post-workout recovery 1,500–2,000 IU D during low energy or menstrual dysfunction	Inadequate vitamin D intake impacts bone health and interferes with calcium absorption. The result? An increased risk of stress fractures, broken bones, and muscle-related injuries.	Fortified cow's/plant-based milk, salmon, tuna, cheese, egg yolks, mushrooms, fortified cereal
VITAMIN K (PHYLLOQUINONE AND MENAQUINONE)	Vitamin K comes in multiple forms with vitamin K_1 (phylloquinone) and vitamin K_2 (menaquinone) being most relevant to health and performance. Phylloquinone is primarily responsible for blood clotting, while menaquinone is critical to bone health and cell growth, and helps improve maximum cardiac output and therefore performance.	90 mcg	Vitamin K deficiency can contribute to an increased risk for bleeding and poor bone health. Given the potential for K_2 to improve performance and prevent osteoporosis, you'd be wise to, at the very least, consume an adequate intake.	Fermented foods (natto), dark green leafy vegetables (collard greens, turnip greens, kale), vegetable oils

MICRONUTRIENTS AND THE FOODS TO CHOOSE

Nutrient	What It Does (Function)	How Much Is Needed Each Day	Possible Effects of a Deficiency	Find It In
VITAMIN C (ASCORBIC ACID)	Just as the name implies, ascorbic acid helps the body to *absorb* iron. A powerful antioxidant, this water-soluble vitamin helps fend off stressors known as free radicals. Vitamin C is also essential for the production of collagen, connective tissue that aids in workout recovery and healthy skin.	75 mg 85 mg: pregnancy 120 mg: lactation	A lack of vitamin C may result in premature fatigue, poor athletic recovery, and poor wound healing, and may impact iron absorption, leading to deficiency.	Oranges, grapefruit, bell peppers, kiwifruit, strawberries, cantaloupe, potatoes, tomatoes
COBALAMIN (VITAMIN B$_{12}$)	This B vitamin is important for healthy blood and nerve cells, both of which impact energy levels and muscle function. This nutrient also helps the body to create DNA, the genetic building blocks of the cells. Vegetarians may struggle to get enough of this nutrient.	2.4 mcg 2.6 mcg: pregnancy 2.8 mcg: lactation	Vitamin B$_{12}$ deficiency accumulates over time, with symptoms lagging. Deficiency can lead to feelings of fatigue, weakness, skin paleness, and poor appetite. All of these are symptoms of pernicious anemia.	Eggs, poultry, fish, red meat, dairy, clams, nutritional yeast, fortified cereal, yogurt
FOLATE	This B vitamin is important for red blood cell production, a key component of oxygen delivery to the muscles. For women of reproductive age, this nutrient is also important for the creation of genetic material and the prevention of neural tube defects during pregnancy.	400 mcg Recommendations range from 600 to 1,000 mcg before conception and throughout pregnancy.	Low folate levels may result in symptoms of fatigue, weakness, shortness of breath, irregular heartbeat, a struggle to focus, and abnormally large red blood cells, thus megaloblastic anemia. Before and during pregnancy, ask your doctor how much to take, as recommendations vary.	Dark leafy greens, asparagus, brussels sprouts, orange juice, nuts, beans, peas, avocados

MICRONUTRIENTS AND THE FOODS TO CHOOSE

Nutrient	What It Does (Function)	How Much Is Needed Each Day	Possible Effects of a Deficiency	Find It In
THIAMINE (VITAMIN B1)	This B vitamin helps your body metabolize foods you fuel with—especially carbohydrate—impacting energy levels and performance. Cells that support muscle growth and assist in tissue repair will reap the benefits of this nutrient.	1.1 mg 1.4 mg: pregnancy and lactation	Inadequate intake of thiamine may lead to muscle weakness, a decrease in appetite, a struggle to gain weight, and the inability to focus.	Whole grains, fortified breads, pasta, rice, pork, fish, legumes, nuts, seeds
RIBOFLAVIN (VITAMIN B2)	Like thiamine, this B vitamin helps food become fuel. This nutrient is involved in glycolysis, the citric acid cycle, and more. The cells involved in muscle growth and tissue repair will reap the benefits of this nutrient. Vegetarians may struggle to get enough of this nutrient.	1.1 mg 1.4 mg: pregnancy 1.6 mg: lactation	Inadequate intake of riboflavin may result in dry/cracked skin, hormone imbalance, hair loss, or even fatigue.	Instant oats, yogurt, mushrooms, almonds, cow's milk, fortified cereal and bread
VITAMIN B6	This B vitamin also plays a big role in turning food into fuel. Vitamin B6 assists with the breakdown and creation of new proteins for muscle gains in the body, as well as supporting immune function.	1.3 mg 1.9 mg: pregnancy 2.0 mg: lactation	Inadequate intake of vitamin B6 may result in poor skin health, a weakened immune system, a lack of energy, and difficulty focusing.	Potatoes, poultry, chickpeas, tuna, salmon, bananas, marinara sauce
MINERALS				
IRON	Iron is essential for athletic performance, as it helps the body create hemoglobin and myoglobin, red blood cells that carry oxygen throughout the body and muscles. Without adequate oxygen, the muscles struggle to move and contract.	18 mg 27 mg: pregnancy and lactation	One of the most common nutrient deficiencies among female endurance athletes, iron deficiency symptoms may include: pale skin, brittle hands, delayed recovery time, increased muscle soreness, lack of energy, difficulty concentrating, fatigue, cravings for ice, and cold hands and feet.	Red meat, poultry, kidney beans, spinach, lentils, peas, nuts, raisins

MICRONUTRIENTS AND THE FOODS TO CHOOSE

Nutrient	What It Does (Function)	How Much Is Needed Each Day	Possible Effects of a Deficiency	Find It In
CALCIUM	Critical for strong and healthy bones, as well as aiding muscle contraction and hormone regulation.	1,000 mg 1,000 mg: pregnancy and lactation (increase to 1,300 mg for teen pregnancy) 1,500 mg: low energy or menstrual dysfunction	Calcium deficiency creates an increased risk of stress fractures and broken bones. Left untreated, it may lead to low bone mass (osteopenia) or brittle bone structure (osteoporosis). During times of low energy and menstrual dysfunction, increase intake.	Cheese, yogurt, cow's/plant-based milk, dark leafy greens, canned sardines with bones, fortified grains and juices
POTASSIUM	An electrolyte, potassium helps muscles contract and keeps your heart pumping. Potassium supports most functions in the body, with an important one for athletic performance being the maintenance of fluid/hydration status alongside sodium.	2,600 mg 2,900 mg: pregnancy 2,800 mg: lactation DV: 4,700 mg (daily value is higher, as other numbers relect a baseline, adequate intake rather than what may be optimal)	Insufficient potassium can result in decreased athletic performance due to muscle weakness, poor muscle contraction, muscle cramping, fatigue, elevated blood pressure, and decreased calcium stores in bones.	Bananas, prunes, dried apricots, raisins, dates, coconut water, potatoes, squash, broccoli, cow's milk, yogurt, lentils
IODINE	Iodine is famous for its role in producing the thyroid hormones needed for many functions in the body, including metabolism and protein synthesis.	150 mcg 220 mcg: pregnancy 290 mcg: lactation	Iodine deficiency may lead to thyroid hypofunction as well as a lack of focus or ability to think clearly.	Cod, tuna, shrimp, yogurt, cheese, milk, iodized salt
ZINC	Zinc helps prevent inflammation and supports the immune system as it works to fight off invaders. Both protein and DNA rely on zinc in order to be created in the body, impacting skin health and wound healing.	8 mg 11 mg: pregnancy 12 mg: lactation 30–40 mg during PMS to combat fatigue and inflammation	Insufficient intake of zinc may result in delayed wound healing, a loss of taste and appetite, and undesired weight loss.	Oysters, red meat, crab, lobster, fortified cereal, legumes, nuts, whole grain bread

MICRONUTRIENTS AND THE FOODS TO CHOOSE

Nutrient	What It Does (Function)	How Much Is Needed Each Day	Possible Effects of a Deficiency	Find It In
MAGNESIUM	Magnesium supports bone health and muscle function, and plays a role in several metabolic processes required for exercise, controlling blood sugar and blood pressure, electrolyte balance, and neuromuscular coordination.	310† mg 350† mg: pregnancy 310† mg: lactation 250 mg supplementation during PMS phase †RDA for age nineteen to thirty. Increase by 10 mg for those over thirty.	Magnesium deficiency may result in a poor appetite, feelings of tiredness, and muscle weakness.	Nuts, legumes, spinach, yogurt, milk, fortified cereal
SELENIUM	This nutrient is mainly stored in the muscles and acts as an antioxidant, helping the body to fight off invaders looking to attack after a heavy bout of exercise.	55 mcg 60 mcg: pregnancy 70 mcg: lactation	While uncommon, selenium deficiency may lead to pain in the joints, swelling, and heart issues.	Nuts, tuna, shrimp, turkey, cottage cheese, brown rice, eggs, oatmeal, whole wheat bread
CHOLINE	Essential for synthesis of cell membranes and plays a role in nerve transmission and brain health, possibly fat metabolism. During pregnancy, it supports the development of the baby's brain and spinal cord.	425 mg 450 mg: pregnancy 550 mg: lactation	Deficiency is uncommon, and exercise does not appear to increase needs. Decreased stores are associated with increased inflammatory markers and a risk of cardiovascular disease.	Beef liver, eggs, fish, nuts, cauliflower, broccoli

What About Supplements?
The Role of Vitamins, Minerals, and Ergogenic Aids in a Healthy Diet

Akin to the eternal question of how many calories an individual should eat, I'm often asked, "Do I need to take a multivitamin?" My answer is, you probably should. Adequate intake of nutrients deemed "essential" is critical for health, growth, and development; healthy aging; and well-being across the life span. But despite a barrage of public health recommendations and extensive media coverage of the health benefits associated with eating a colorful, varied diet, most Americans fail miserably in this department. For example, the vegetables most frequently consumed in the United States are potatoes and tomatoes, with french fries and pizza sauce being the most common sources.

Americans fall below the recommended intake of several essential nutrients—vitamins A, D, E, and K; vitamin C; magnesium; and calcium—despite an abundant supply of nutrient-dense foods available to fill the gap. So while some people don't *need* more of each and *every* nutrient included in a multivitamin, I view these supplements as cheap insurance.

Approximately half of U.S. adults take one or more supplements daily. Roughly 65 percent of female collegiate varsity athletes report consuming supplements, with multivitamins being the most common supplements used by both male and female student-athletes and women more likely to consume vitamin C, iron, calcium, and magnesium.

The exact effects of supplementation on female health and performance remain unclear, with generalized data findings extrapolated to women. To date, the vast majority of studies focusing on ergogenic aids—supplements that increase the capacity for physical or mental performance—revolve around male athletes, even though women respond differently to many of these aids. A few popular supplements have begun to be examined, but there is certainly more work to be done.

Pro Tips for Optimizing Micronutrient Supplementation

Just as there's an art to nailing the when and what of optimal fueling, the same goes for many supplements. To get the optimal effect and absorption from your dietary supplements, you'll want to consider the form to take as well as the combinations and timing. The chart on the following page is adapted from advice from Marie Spano, one of the country's leading sports nutritionists; she works with professional sports teams as well as individuals ranging from youth to pro athletes. These are also common supplements and nutrients of concern that I frequently recommend to clients. Keep Spano's tips in mind when supplementing vitamins and minerals and when choosing foods rich in specific nutrients.

Nutrient(s)	Pro Tips
FAT-SOLUBLE VITAMINS A, D, E, K	Improve absorption by consuming alongside a meal that contains fat.
VITAMIN D	Take alongside calcium. Choose a supplement with the active form, D_3 (cholecalciferol).
CALCIUM	Stagger your intake across the day, taking no more than 500 mg at one time. Take calcium carbonate with food, calcium citrate at any time. Do not take at the same time as a multivitamin or an iron or zinc supplement. Do not take with antacids, laxatives, prednisone, antibiotics, or levothyroxine.
IRON	Take on an empty stomach if possible. Consider taking with vitamin C–rich juice or foods but never with milk or caffeine. Do not take at the same time as a multivitamin or a calcium supplement.
MAGNESIUM	Take with or without food. Consider taking before bed (magnesium citrate can be taken anytime, but magnesium glycinate or bisglycinate are preferable for sleep). Do not take with bisphosphonates, antibiotics, diuretics, acid reflux meds, or very high doses of zinc. Do not combine with calcium or dairy.
MULTIVITAMIN	Take with food. Do not take with other individual-nutrient supplements. Avoid taking alongside fiber supplements or medications.
OMEGA-3 (FISH OIL / FLAXSEED)	Take with a meal that contains fat. Consider freezing the capsule to help prevent discomforting "fishy burps." Add 1 gram per day throughout the PMS phase.
FIBER SUPPLEMENTS	While fiber supplements are not a micronutrient, do not take them at the same time as vitamin or protein supplements, as absorption of these nutrients may be negatively impacted.

Pro Tip: Don't neglect your bones. All over the world, the most frequent sufferers of osteoporosis and osteopenia are women. You deposit critical bone mass until the late teenage years and possibly into your twenties. Prioritize foods with bone-building calcium, vitamin D, vitamin K, and magnesium. Avoid bone baddies like smoking and excessive alcohol intake. Soft drinks and excessive caffeine intake can be problematic, so moderation or avoidance is a better choice. If you're experiencing low energy availability or RED-S, it's imperative to address the underlying issues. Stress reactions, stress fractures, and missing your period are huge warning signs that there's something wrong, including the loss of bone density, from which you may never be able to recover.

ERGOGENIC AIDS: PERFORMANCE-ENHANCING SUPPLEMENTS

Supplement	Why to Use	How It Works	How to Use: Timing	How to Use: Dose	Possible Side Effects	Sources
CALCIUM BETA-HYDROXY-BETA-METHYLBUTYRATE (HMB)	Use during heavy training to thwart delayed-onset muscle soreness and possibly lend improvement to VO₂ max and endurance performance metrics as well as strength gains. Use while injured to prevent losses in lean mass.	The metabolite of leucine helps prevent muscle breakdown and promotes muscle protein synthesis.	Split into two 1.5-gram doses; one dose 60 minutes pre-exercise and one within 2 hours post-exercise.	2.5 to 3 grams per day. (Effective dose in literature is 3 grams, but this is based on larger male bodies.)	Poor-tasting supplement but no side effects anticipated.	Supplement with powdered calcium HMB in drink form (Abbott Juven) or free acid form. Present in some foods but not in the efficacious dose needed.
CAFFEINE	Reduces RPE, can improve focus and concentration, may help break down fat stores and mobilize free fatty acids for use during exercise. Use for longer, sustained efforts.	CNS stimulant. Increases blood pressure, heart rate, stomach acid production. During times with more estradiol in the bloodstream, greater impact of caffeine-related side effects but no change in performance.	Blood levels peak 45 to 60 minutes post-ingestion. Max effect can take up to 3 to 4 hours. Use frequently during exercise, as exercise clears caffeine.	2–3 mg/kg/hr during activity. Thwart PMS by consuming across workout.	Jitteriness, insomnia, restlessness, nausea. Moderate intake isn't banned, but excessive levels (greater than 15 mcg/ml in urine or about 500 mg ingested) will result in a positive drug test. At this level, side effects derail performance.	Coffee, tea, soda, pills, gums, shots, select chews, bars, gels

ERGOGENIC AIDS: PERFORMANCE-ENHANCING SUPPLEMENTS

Supplement	Why to Use	How It Works	How to Use: Timing	How to Use: Dose	Possible Side Effects	Sources
CREATINE MONOHYDRATE	Helps muscle cells produce energy during strength- and power-based, HIIT activities; bursts lasting less than 10 seconds which would tax the phosphocreatine system. Short-term and long-term supplementation enhances muscular strength and power and other measures of anaerobic and aerobic exercise performance, with minimal effects on body composition.	Found in animal proteins and stored in the skeletal muscle. Supplementation increases phosphocreatine stores up to 20 percent. Supplementation by females tends to show greater relative improvements. Evolving research points to positive impact on mood and cognition as well as brain health, augmenting antidepressant effects.	More potential TBD: may be of particular importance during menses, pregnancy, postpartum, pre- and postmenopause.	Load with 0.3 grams per kilogram per day for 5–7 days; or use a routine daily dose (3 to 5 grams) for 4 weeks. During times of recovery from injury, 10 grams per day for 2 weeks, decrease to 5 grams per day for next 4 to 6 weeks.	Potential for GI distress, attenuation in natural productions, concern with renal and kidney impact. Documentation of side effects is lacking; research suggests clear record of safety when used as recommended. Worried about weight gain? Don't be.	Powdered supplement
BETA-ALANINE	Improves exercise performance in exercises lasting 60 to 240 seconds (sprints, fast finishes); helps muscle fiber firing rates and recovery; effective in exercises lasting longer but to a lesser magnitude.	Precursor to carnosine, which acts as a pH buffer during exercise. Females have lower levels of carnosine and thus experience greater levels of muscle carnosine after beta-alanine supplementation.		3.2–6.4 grams per day. Start at lower dosage or separate into two smaller doses per day to thwart paresthesia.	Paresthesia: numbing in feet, hands, and face, which is not dangerous but an unusual sensation. Start with a lower dose and increase as tolerated.	Capsules, supplements, often found in pre-workout ergogenic aids

ERGOGENIC AIDS: PERFORMANCE-ENHANCING SUPPLEMENTS

Supplement	Why to Use	How It Works	How to Use: Timing	How to Use: Dose	Possible Side Effects	Sources
BRANCHED-CHAIN AMINO ACIDS (BCAA)	BCAA supplementation before and after exercise has beneficial effects, decreasing exercise-induced muscle damage and promoting muscle protein synthesis. Use of BCAAs may attenuate exercise-induced muscle damage that causes delayed-onset muscle soreness.	The amino acids leucine, isoleucine, and valine are involved in specific biochemical muscle processes. Consumption of BCAAs while exercising in the heat has been shown to prolong moderate exercise performance.	Pre-workout during PMS phase to decrease negative impact of estrogen-progesterone on CNS. Post-workout 2 to 3 grams (within 30 grams whey protein powder or on own) to fend off injury.	5–7 grams	Besides the taste, and occasional GI effects, there are few if any significant side effects from BCAA supplementation.	Powdered supplement, naturally occurring in select sources of protein

PART 2

BUILD THE STRUCTURE

MAKE IT MINDFUL: LIFE HACKS TO FIGHT FOOD TRIGGERS AND EMOTIONAL EATING

You know the *what*, the *why*, and (will soon be introduced to) the *when* behind optimal nutrition, so where's the missing link? Why is it so difficult for so many of us to make consistently healthy choices? Regardless of athletic ability, our choices are influenced by access, economics, and taste preferences. But there's more to the story. Emotions commonly rule the plate. For better or worse, some of us are more emotionally connected to foods. Across interviews with countless athletes, there appears to be a divide between perception of food as a helpful tool or else a necessary evil. Those who view food as supportive and power for performance navigate a less rocky path. Deena Kastor is a world-class runner and shining example of how to view food in a positive light.

CHANGE YOUR PERSPECTIVE TO CHANGE YOUR PERFORMANCE

When asked how she stayed friends with food, Deena Kastor, an Olympian world record holder, said she mindfully considers food not as an enemy but as an ally and powerful tool.

Kastor began to read about nutrition and learned that optimal fuel could aid performance. The right nutrients could differentiate her performance from that of others. Her positive mindset and perspective prompted her to consider how almost every food brings purpose and potential. Kastor has worked to maintain this positive perspective, fueling strategically with high-quality nutrition across her career. As an American record holder, Olympic medalist, and eight-time national cross-country champion, obviously she's doing something right!

Change isn't always quick and easy. Amanda Carlson-Phillips is a sports dietitian with EXOS, a company that focuses on proactive health and performance for elite athletes. She explains: "The emotional connection to food is not gender or sport agnostic—it really is a human thing. When athletes understand this emotional connection and tune into it, performance comes to life." Having worked with elite athletes over a period of many years, Carlson-Phillips has observed countless on-off approaches to nutrition. "Athletes will focus and adapt their fueling and dial it in for a period, and then they completely go the other direction in the off-season." Carlson-Phillips adds this cyclical approach presents challenges to health; it's a poor habit that can ultimately impede recovery and forestall improvements in strength and power. "We encourage athletes to aim for consistency and trend toward an approach that has them optimally fueling as their default fueling strategy."

DEAR YOUNGER, HUNGRY ME: DEENA KASTOR

As one of the best American distance runners of all time, Deena is the former American record holder in the marathon (2:19:36) and the half-marathon (1:07:34). She is a three-time Olympian, earning a bronze in the 2004 marathon in Athens, and has won the London and Chicago marathons. With wicked fast personal records in the 5,000 (14:51) and 10,000 (30:50), Deena continues to crush records; she holds the American Masters half-marathon and marathon records too. One of the most gracious and engaging people you will ever encounter, Deena attributes much of her success to the power of positive thinking and a sense of gratitude, and she details this perspective throughout the pages of her bestselling book *Let Your Mind Run*. Not one to sit still, Deena trains with the Mammoth Track Club, coached by her husband, Andrew Kastor, and is a role model for her daughter, Piper. During her career, Deena has looked to running to challenge her and help her power through adversity. She's sought food as fuel, to provide purposeful support and power across challenges and miles. Here I share her encouraging words and uplifting perspective with you.

Dear Younger, Hungry Deena,

Pause everything. Go into the kitchen and have fun stirring up something fabulous. As you cook, think about what you want out of the meal. Satisfaction? Greater endurance? Joy? Strength for an upcoming workout? Your intention is strong so use it to your advantage.

As you eat, enjoy the labor of love you are feeding yourself. You deserve the best ingredients, cooked or prepared with great purpose, and eaten with the utmost of pleasure. Once you can give yourself this gift, invite people around the table and share the gift of good food with them. In the future, your table will be big and full of friends and laughter.

Other than an unexplored running trail, this will be your favorite place on earth. Once a good meal is done and the plates are cleared, you are fueled to chase all that you dream of.

Love,
Fulfilled Deena

WORKING TOWARD CHANGE

But how to find consistency and strategic eating when you're often on an emotional roller coaster? Like it or not, human beings are rarely rational when it comes to food. We don't purchase, prepare, and consume foods based solely on what we need to survive. The art of eating is not as simple as balancing nutrient-dense calories in with metabolic cost of calories out. Instead we live in a world where hunger and appetite are intertwined and emotional eating is prevalent.

Think through the last time you craved a home-cooked meal while lonely (there's a reason it's called *comfort food*), snacked instead of checking off some items on the to-do list (guilty!), or numbed a stressful day with ice cream. Don't be too hard on yourself; humans are biologically wired to be highly emotional beings. Our hormones have a significant influence on our day-to-day decision-making, with fluctuations throughout each cycle, making some days even more emotionally driven. Thus, emotions and hormones have a direct impact on calorie intake and choices. Instead of responding to hunger, we often eat to numb feelings, diminish boredom, and avoid discomfort.

So stop blaming yourself for turning to calories to cope rather than engaging in mindful consumption. You've got lots of (great) company in your quest to seek a tasty and immediate solution to every discomfort. There's science behind this: many of the foods we seek out when stressed contain ingredients—primarily sugars—that have been shown to light up the same areas of the brain as cocaine and a host of other illicit drugs. Such foods trigger a similar post-consumption euphoria but also lead to withdrawal symptoms and cravings after the fact. And over time, the hypothesis goes, we become desensitized to the effects, therefore seeking more and more of the "good stuff" to increase the release of dopamine, the neurotransmitter known to play a role in feelings of pleasure, given the part it plays in reward-motivated behavior. However, this euphoria will wane, leaving you to deal with the real task at hand.

Pro Tip: When you are handed a day from hell and are tempted to cope with food, pause. Are you truly hungry or simply looking to distract yourself? Once the momentary pleasure or numbness you expect from that sometimes food fades, you'll be left to deal with the original distress, now compounded by the guilt you're likely to experience as well as the stress, the to-do list, and the emotions that remain. When you look at it like this, it's probably easier to confront the distress from the get-go.

Life Hacks to Fight Emotional Eating

LIFE HACK 1: Differentiate between hunger and appetite. Ask yourself, could the urge to eat be driven by something other than physical hunger? Write down your urges and feelings and rank your level of physical hunger and that of emotional discomfort on scales of 1 to 10. Is there a pattern driving your choices? For example, your journal may show that after every team practice, you either binge eat or have no appetite at all. By logging your emotions and your response to them, you may discover your diet is driven not by hunger but by needing a way to cope with stress.

LIFE HACK 2: Set a timer. You just ate, but if you're like my kids, you're "hungry" again. Set a timer for 20 minutes. Take a walk, call a friend, play the piano. Find an activity that occupies your hands and distracts you. A 20-minute time gap is purposeful; it gives you time to consider whether you are experiencing true hunger, and it removes you from the situation should the pull be emotional rather than an actual need for calories.

LIFE HACK 3: Shut it down. You've finished dinner, smartly fueled throughout your day, met your macros, and answered the call of hunger. It's time to close the kitchen. Store food out of sight, out of mind. Use baskets or opaque containers, or even hide food behind cabinet doors (locked if you must). Unless you've got an early long workout looming, there's likely no need to top off the tank before bed.

LIFE HACK 4: Set small goals. A little goes a long way when it comes to making a permanent change. Instead of taking on too much at once, which can lead to your feeling overwhelmed and defeated, choose one or two small changes you're confident you can make and consistently carry out every day.

LIFE HACK 5: Find a new reward. You're definitely not alone if you're tempted to reward long runs and intense workouts with food. The mindset that you just burned X calories so you deserve the treat is pervasive. This practice sets you up for eating more calories than you expended and sets a dangerous precedent of linking food with behavior. Instead, link your hard work to something calorie free and less fleeting. New shoes after 400 miles or a massage after a killer workout is a great place to start.

LIFE HACK 6: Invoke the celery rule. Remember when you were a child and you asked for a snack (even though you had just eaten)? Your caregiver, probably still cleaning up the recent meal and realizing you couldn't be hungry, said something along the lines of "If you're hungry, you can have some celery." This rule serves to help you distinguish hunger from craving. If you're hungry, grab something healthy, like celery. If only dessert will do, see other Life Hacks.

LIFE HACK 7: Revamp your environment. Shelves packed with junk food increase the likelihood you'll consume said junk foods. So stop buying the junk foods. Eating in front of the TV prompts appetite every time you sit down to watch. Eat at the table instead. Scrolling social media will convince you you're out of shape, underperforming, worthless. Close the account, delete the app, stop subjecting yourself to the bull.

THE MOST IMPORTANT LIFE HACK: Cut yourself a break. You'll hear the sage advice to *be kind to yourself* echoed by every single expert in these pages. Begin by treating yourself the way you would a friend who is striving to make changes for the better. You would be supportive, kind, gentle, and encouraging. We women are often guilty of being our own harshest critic, full of thoughts that undermine us rather than help us rise. Raise yourself up rather than beating yourself down. The simple fact that you are reading this book, changing the way you think about food and self, means that you are already rising to the challenge of building a better you.

DEAR YOUNGER, HUNGRY ME: MOLLY SEIDEL

What would it be like to win a bronze Olympic medal in only your third attempt at the distance? Would you think yourself gifted (yes) or would you embrace the fact that countless hard effort and miles, not to mention passion and dedication, paid off? With no BS about her, Molly Seidel is a top American distance runner who thrilled the world at the Tokyo Olympics in one of her first attempts at the distance. But her medal came after years of pushing her limits. She won the high school Foot Locker Cross Country Championships, was an all-American at Notre Dame, NCAA D1 champion in cross-country, an indoor track and field winner (3,000 and 5,000 meters), an outdoor 10,000-meter champion, and a six-time Atlantic Coast Conference champion. The hurdles Molly faced along the way to each of these podiums were many. A victim of countless injuries and setbacks while navigating mental health needs, she's worked as hard to heal and "unpack" as she has to win medals and achievements. Molly shares real and raw experiences, offering a refreshing and often relatable journey. You're sure to appreciate her transparent and honest nature and join in my gratitude for her selfless sharing of her journey across dark days and into the light of recovery, healing, and of course winning.

Dear Younger, Hungry Molly circa 2008,

You're just starting out in this whole running thing. It's your first season of high school cross-country, and you've shown a lot of talent but are wondering how far this could take you. You don't know it right now, but this is going to be so much harder than you think it will be, but it will be so incredibly worth it. This sport will break your heart a million times. It'll hurt your body, push you mentally further than you ever thought you could go, and make you question why you do it. But you will love what you do so deeply, to the degree where you could never imagine doing anything else. The lowest of lows will be matched by the highest of highs. But those highs won't be possible unless you are healthy.

The best piece of advice I can give you as you start down this road is to listen to your body. In every sense, from eating to training to just simply living.

First off, if you are hungry, then eat. Simple as that. Training takes an enormous amount of energy and calories, and you simply can't succeed in the sport without properly fueling. If you aren't giving your body the raw materials it needs, it'll be able to last for a while but is eventually going to shut you down as it works to preserve itself. Hunger isn't something you should fight; it's your body's way of telling you it needs nutrition.

Your body is incredibly smart, and I've found that when I consume a high-quality nutritious diet, then my cravings usually reflect the actual needs of my body. If I crave meat, then I probably need more protein or iron. Craving carbs means my glycogen stores are depleted and need to be restocked before the next training session. Chocolate cravings are usually a sign my period is about to hit, so I treat myself.

Trying to deny or restrict ultimately leads to nutrient deficiencies, or worse, the binging and purging behaviors you'll face in college. When you fight your body, you can hold out only so long; it'll find a way to shut you down through either exhaustion or injury until you finally give it what it needs. So stop fighting and learn to accept the needs of your body, and it'll reward you with health and performance for years.

Second point: when it comes to your mental health, listen to what your body is telling you. Over the course of your career you are going to face a number of mental health struggles, mainly OCD, anxiety, and depression. You'll find ways to channel these into strengths in running; however, you will also face a seemingly disproportionate amount of burnout compared to your peers as you try to push past the times your mind tells you it needs a break.

Finally, have faith that your body will tell you what it needs and will lead you in the right direction. You will struggle for years trying to fit your body into a box of what it "should" look like or how an elite runner is "supposed" to train. Only when you start training in a sustainable way will you be able to find actual success and happiness in this sport. When you work with your body rather than against it, resting when it tells you to rest and pushing when it says to push, then you can achieve more than you ever thought possible.

So good luck, freshman year Molly. You've got a wild ride ahead of you, and enjoy every wonderful, painful, crazy moment of it.

REACHING FOR BETTER:
AN EXERCISE IN HABIT BUILDING

S till struggling to put the knowledge of the types and amounts of foods to eat into practice? *Nutrition is a science, but eating is an emotion.* Or maybe you know it takes sweat equity, training, and dedication to hit the next level of performance but still can't find the time or desire to hit the gym? Setting goals, building habits, and reaching out for help might be in order.

START WITH SECURING SOME SUPPORT

Listen, ladies. If you want to march confidently toward your goals, support along the way will keep you on course and make you love every step. You need someone to shout encouragement, keep you motivated and accountable. What you don't need is someone who's not in your corner. You don't need someone who complains that your Netflix marathons have shifted to real marathons. Or who whines when you no longer binge drink with them or bury your sorrows in sweets.

When you decide to reach for better, your likelihood of success improves when those who matter most to you are supportive. Ready to get everyone on board? This practical approach and worksheet can help make it all possible.

State your case: Share your goal, explain your why, and dig deep. Spend time in self-reflection and write down the intricacies of your goal and why it's important. Then set aside time for a compelling conversation. Remember, just because you want to build your best self doesn't necessarily mean you want to go it alone, so include others when it's appropriate so they too can benefit from better days ahead.

Write it down:

My goal is SMART (specific, measurable, amazing, realistic, time bound): _____

_____

Here's why it matters: _____

I plan to begin chasing this goal on _____ *and reach the finish*
line on _____.

Here's what you can expect in return (how you envision changing or how your self-improvements benefit the group or even what you'll do in return for their help):

_____

Be clear about what's required: Changing for the better takes work. And removing obstacles in your path can get tricky. Prepare your tribe for some adjustments, and be clear about the types of changes and commitments you think will be needed to bring this goal to life.

Here's what it will take to bring this goal to life: 1. _____
2. _____ *3.* _____

Changes you can expect will include (i.e., how your support system will be impacted):

_____

Ask for help already! Why is it so damn hard to ask for help? Why are women more prone to the "do it all" martyr mentality? Start with a strong will, stepping up and clearly articulating the help you'll need and why their support is critical, and for just a split second, let someone else carry the weight of the world.

I can't/won't/don't want to go this alone because _____

_____

I'm coming to you for help. Here's what I need: _____

_____

Stay the course. During times of doubt and pushback, remember your why. There's a reason you started working to create a new outlook and a new outcome. Self-reflection can help you stay motivated should things get tough. Accept that not everyone will be thrilled or embrace the better you. Don't let these vibes bring you down. Remember, you fought to get started, you've worked to build a better you. Don't let anyone rain on your parade.

There's a chance I'll experience pushback. Possible obstacles might be _____

_____

Here's what I'll do to stay focused: _____

_____

Here are some healthy ways to cope when needed: _____

_____

Here's what I'll do to quiet the critics: _____

_____

PRACTICE MAKES PERFECT: A REAL-LIFE EXAMPLE

I've used this technique multiple times, and here's an example to bring the act of securing support to life:

State your case:

My goal is: **to run a marathon.**

Here's why it's important to me: **I'm at my happiest and best self when running, and I thrive while chasing a dream and challenging myself. Running makes me a better wife, friend, and mom.**

Here's what you can expect (in return): **I'm always in a better mood after I work out and more motivated to do my best work. I know training takes a lot of time, but I want to be a healthy and fit role model and show our kids the traits of consistency and dedication.**

Be clear about what's required:

This is going to take work. Here's what I think that looks like: **Two early morning runs each week and one long run on Sundays. Sixteen weeks of training building from 20 miles to 45 miles per week. The race takes place the first week in November and will require a plane ticket and a hotel room.**

Ask for help:

I can't do this alone. To bring this goal to life, here's what I need: **Can you please be in charge during my morning runs before school, making sure everyone has a lunch and is wearing clean clothes? When I'm done with my run, I'll wash your workout clothes (alongside mine) and make your life a little easier too. And since I'll be running long on days I usually do the grocery shopping, can you** *please help? And can you not bring home bulk bags of candy? I get so hungry and tired during training, and kiddie mix is my Achilles' heel!*

Stay the course:

*There's a chance I'll experience pushback. I'll stay focused by **referring to my sixteen-week plan and realizing that one missed run does not derail a race.***

*Here's what I'll do to cope: **If I get injured, I'll cross-train at the YMCA pool, use the time to strength-train, or I'll catch up on laundry.***

*Here's what I'll do to quiet the critics: **Consistent training and dedication to fueling will keep me strong and ready to perform.***

KITCHEN ESSENTIALS

A helpful and healthy habit to have is knowing your way around the kitchen. Fortunately, you don't have to be the next Julia Child in order to cook and eat healthily. You just need to master a few skills and have the right tools at hand. What's deemed an "essential" tool is as varied as the cooks themselves. If you haven't (yet) gotten comfortable in the kitchen or if you're now at a place in your life when it's time to prioritize these tools, the list below is a great starting point. Dana Angelo White is a registered dietitian, a certified athletic trainer, the nutrition expert for FoodNetwork.com, the sports food and nutrition expert at Quinnipiac University, a rock-star mom of three, and the author of nine books, including *DASH Diet Meal Prep for Beginners* and *Healthy, Quick & Easy College Cookbook*. She sounded in with some of her basic kitchen must-haves.

POTS, PANS, and BAKEWARE

Dutch Oven

Best uses: slow-cooking, braising, roasting, stewing

What to look for: enameled cast iron to maintain an even and consistent heat, suitable for both stovetop and oven use; 4½–5½ quarts (or more if you're feeding a crowd) is most versatile

Price range: $150–$400 (pick a good one and it will last a lifetime)

Expert pick: Le Creuset Dutch Oven

Cast-Iron Skillet

Best uses: baking, sautéing, searing, frying

What to look for: preseasoned, thick bottom with straight sides, comfortable handle

Price range: $25–$150

Expert pick: Lodge Cast-Iron Skillet

Nonstick Skillet or Fry pan

Best uses: sautéing, frying, searing with or without oil

What to look for: pan that's 10 to 12 inches in diameter with a thick bottom for durability and for even heat distribution; dark, nonstick surface that's PFOA free and won't chip or flake

Price range: $40–$180

Expert pick: Le Creuset Nonstick Fry Pan

Saucepan

Best uses: boiling, steaming, making sauces and soups

What to look for: multiple sizes (I find I use my 2-quart and 4-quart pots most often), stainless-steel material, with an easy-to-grip handle and a "helping handle" for an extra grab point

Price range: $60–$300

Expert pick: All-Clad d5 Stainless-Steel Saucepan, 2 quart

Rimmed Baking Sheet (Jelly Roll Pan)

Best uses: one-pan meals, roasting, baking

What to look for: light-colored surface that browns evenly, high sides, sturdy but lightweight

Price range: $15–$40 (for a half sheet)

Expert pick: Nordic Ware Baker's Half Sheet

KNIVES and HAND TOOLS

CHEF'S KNIFE

Best uses: chopping, dicing, mincing

What to look for: thin 8-inch blade made from high-carbon stainless steel or Damascus steel

Price range: $25–$200

Expert picks: Victorinox Fibrox Pro 8-Inch Chef's Knife

PARING KNIFE

Best uses: slicing, peeling, chopping

What to look for: 3- to 4-inch blade that's sharp, lightweight, and slightly flexible with a secure handle

Price range: $10–$20

Expert pick: Colori Titanium Paring Knife

SERRATED KNIFE

Best uses: slicing breads, baked goods, smooth-skinned fruits and vegetables, or meat

What to look for: 10-inch blade with fewer broader, deeper pointed serrations, comfortable easy-to-grip handle of medium weight

Price range: $20–$125

Expert picks: Global Classic 6-Inch Serrated Utility Knife or Wüsthof Classic 10-Inch Double-Serrated Bread Knife

VEGETABLE PEELER

Best uses: peeling vegetables (obviously) as well as fruits and potatoes; also
   great for peeling thin slices of cheese off blocks
What to look for: sturdy and sharp carbon blade, adequate space between peeler
   and blade to prevent jamming
Price range: $3–$10
Expert picks: OXO Good Grips Swivel Peeler

OTHER TOOLS

MASON JARS

Best uses: smoothies, salads, salad dressing, cold storage
What to look for: 8- to 16-ounce size with lid
Price range: $10–$20 per dozen
Expert pick: Ball Wide Mouth Pint Glass Mason Jars

MEASURING CUPS—LIQUID AND DRY

Best uses: portion control, precise measurements for baking and
   cooking
What to look for:
   Dry: easy-to-read measurement markings, stack and store neatly, handles
      flush with cup, made of heavy-gauge stainless steel, dishwasher safe
   Liquid: crisp markings in ¼ and ⅓ cup increments, heatproof,
      microwavable, glass
Price range: $5–$45
Expert pick: OXO Good Grips Stainless-Steel Measuring Cups Set (dry), Pyrex
   1- and 2-cup measuring cups (liquid)

MEASURING SPOONS

Best uses: precise measuring of small amounts of ingredients

What to look for: easy-to-read measurement markings, stack and store neatly, long handle that is flush with rim of bowl, elongated bowls that can fit inside spice jars

Price range: $10–$20

Expert pick: Le Creuset Stainless-Steel Measuring Spoons

SALAD SPINNER

Best uses: cleaning and storing lettuce, chopped vegetables and fruit

What to look for: ergonomic and easy-to-operate lid/handle, flat (or collapsible) lid for easy storage

Price range: $30–$60

Expert pick: OXO Good Grips Stainless-Steel Salad Spinner

STACKED MIXING BOWLS

Best uses: mixing, meal prep

What to look for: lightweight, easy to handle, tempered glass or stainless steel, dishwasher safe

Price range: $15–$40

Expert pick: OXO Good Grips Three-Piece Stainless-Steel Mixing Bowl Set

SMALL APPLIANCES

HIGH-POWERED BLENDER

Best uses: smoothies, soups, sauces, grain flours

What to look for: proper-size canister for your needs, mix of straight and serrated blades at varying angles, heavy base for stability

Price range: $300–$400

Expert pick: Vitamix, Blendtec

Electric Pressure Cooker

Best uses: quick meals, stews, chili, rice, hard-cooked eggs

What to look for: easy-to-read pressure indicator, intuitive control panel with programmable timer and warning mode; small countertop footprint

Price range: $120–$140

Expert pick: Instant Pot Duo Plus 6 Quart 9-in-1

Air Fryer

Best uses: fish, potatoes, egg rolls, chicken wings/homemade nuggets

What to look for: a unit that isn't too bulky but has a good-size inner basket; a digital control panel is ideal

Price range: $75–$150

Expert pick: Bella or Kyvol

MEAL PREP 101: THE LIFE HACK YOU NEED NOW

Meal prepping, which involves only a small investment of time up front, yields a huge payoff. Not only will you have an easier week ahead, but you'll also fuel your most important goals with the nutrition you need. Here's a quick and simple crash course in meal prepping, including some ideas you'll quickly put into practice.

PLAN AROUND YOUR GOALS

Good food choices often get sidelined when life is hectic. Mindless eating and surrendering to temptation (hello, drive-through) can quickly become the new norm in a busy schedule.

Just like anything worth having, meal prep takes work. However, the social media version of it (countless rows of picture-perfect containers) isn't required. The art of meal prep can be incredibly simple.

Getting Started

STEP 1: THERE'S NO PREP WITHOUT THE PLAN.

As Benjamin Franklin put it, "Success is the residue of planning." Who knew he was a meal prepper? This quote is spot-on. You're better equipped to hit any calorie or macro- and micronutrient targets with well-designed meals.

So grab your calendar and look at the week ahead. If you're like most of us, you'll have a mix of meal occasions and meals you'll want to prep for. Before you start thinking food, think bigger picture.

- ▸ What are *all* the typical meals in your day? People often forget about planning for snacks, but these small bites add up to a big part of your menu.
- ▸ What are your biggest meal struggles? Is it a healthy dinner option that gets pushed aside at the end of a long day when you're fatigued and famished and order takeout?
- ▸ Are your on-the-go daily lunches adding up in cost and unhealthy choices?

As your weekly picture emerges, you'll see where meal planning can help. If you need to start small with only one planned mealtime for the week, this is a great first step we can build on later.

Yes, life is busy, time is tight, and "convenient" options may seem appealing in the moment, but they could be setting you back. In her book *DASH Diet Meal Prep for Beginners*, Dana Angelo White notes: "When you don't have a plan and are hungry, the last-minute food options available aren't usually your first—or best—choice. Meal planning can help you stay on track with your health goals and make following [your plan] a whole lot easier." Simply put, meal planning is a game changer for living your healthiest life.

STEP 2: MATCH MEALS WITH GOALS.

Your meals are fuel for your current needs and future goals.

If you're injured and repairing, you'll want to plan for enough chicken, veggie burgers, and lean protein for recovery and satiety. If you're in the midst of marathon hell week,

Pro Tip: Time it right: Meal plan when you're calm and motivated to eat for better health and performance. This solid blueprint will keep you grounded and committed to healthy choices even if/when life hits the fan.

Sunday will find you boiling pasta, steaming rice, soaking pre-run oats, and getting those recovery smoothies ready.

Meal prep is one of the best tools to get you closer to your goals without detours. If you need more clarity about the top fuel to choose, check out the Go-To Options for Meal Prep on page 109.

STEP 3: FOLLOW THE RECIPE FOR SUCCESS (FOR EVERYONE).

It's time to get excited about the week ahead, and that means having a meal plan you and your entire family will be eager to try out. I promise it's not impossible!

First, find meals that spark your interest, meet your nutrition goals, and store well. If you need inspiration, countless blogs, social media foodies, and cookbooks exist, all offering amazing recipes. You can't go wrong with a few of my personal favorites from Half-Baked Harvest, America's Test Kitchen, or Cook's Illustrated.

Your own preferences are the easy part. What about the rest of your tribe? It's a challenge to have picky eaters (ahem, please meet my four-year-old) or different dietary needs (like being a plant-based eater in a house full of carnivores) all at a single table. It's totally doable, though.

Once you've got your master plan (including meals and snacks), sketch it out. Before you head to the store, peek in your fridge and cabinets. Based on what you already have (including fresh items like veggies that need to be used up), you can tweak your plan to save some time and money.

STEP 4: NOW IT'S TIME TO SHOP.

Never head to the store (even if it's online!) hungry. It's an invitation for impulse buys, unhealthy choices, and a huge grocery bill.

Here are a few parts of the store you'll spend most of your time in:

Produce (fresh veggies, fruits): You'll save money if you wash, chop, and prep items yourself.

Proteins (meats, eggs, etc.): Meal planning guarantees you'll use these items when they're at their freshest.

Frozen section: Don't be afraid to try out frozen veggies (they're often picked at the peak of their freshness and flash-frozen to lock in nutrients), ready-made meatballs, or other heat-and-eat options if time is tight.

Food containers: Warehouse clubs are often a great source for bulk takeout containers. Look for options that are microwave, freezer, and dishwasher safe. Bonus points for choosing containers that are stackable, BPA free, and reusable.

I personally prefer to pack my to-go smoothies and shakes in leakproof and insulated stainless-steel vacuum jars (my go-to is Hydro Flask Food Jars). If I'm home, I'll just use inexpensive mason jars. For meal prepping, I use high-quality glass containers with tight-sealing lids so I can pop them into the freezer and heat them up later in the microwave or oven.

Whatever containers you choose, make sure you have at least one container for each meal you plan to prep. For most of us, ten containers (five lunches, five dinners) is great for the workweek. You'll also need to pay attention to the size. If you use a large (family-size) container for a personal to-go meal, you'll be more likely to consume larger portions. Instead, choose smaller containers that will satisfy you, without making you need a nap an hour later!

STEP 5: HERE COMES THE FUN (COOKING AND PORTIONS).

Unless you're a meal prep pro who wants to tackle all these steps at once, we recommend staging this process to make it easy when you're new to it and simple to incorporate into a permanent routine.

After you've shopped, use the second day to prep, cook, and store meals. These last three steps take some time, so dedicate some of your Sunday to it, especially if this is your post-long-run rest day, and make it fun by listening to some music or a podcast while you work.

Once all your entrées, sides, or individual ingredients are fully prepared, grab your containers. Portion them evenly to make sure your intake is consistent throughout the week (avoiding the mistake of double protein on Monday and nothing but rice on Friday).

Dana Angelo White cautions that prepped food shouldn't sit out longer than two hours. Refrigerate food within an hour of cooking, cooling it in shallow containers if more efficient cooling is needed. Mark containers with the date the food was prepared, and store them in the coldest part of the fridge, typically in the back on the door hinge side, but make sure leafy greens don't get accidentally frozen. Typically, meals last approximately five days without spoiling. Remember to store frozen foods using an airtight container, and label items with the name of the food, the date frozen, and cooking instructions. If anticipating long-term freezing, seal food with plastic wrap to prevent freezer burn and food waste.

Store It Right

Curious as to how long you can safely store food and have it taste as good as it did on day one? Refer to this chart, adapted from FoodSafety.gov.

Category	Food Specifics	Refrigerator (40°F or below)	Freezer (0°F or below)*
VEGGIE-BASED SALAD	Leaf lettuce with fresh vegetable toppings	3 days	Freezing not recommended
PROTEIN-BASED SALAD	Egg, chicken, ham, tuna, bean salad	3 to 4 days	Freezing not recommended
PROCESSED MEAT—DELI MEAT, BACON, SAUSAGE	Deli meat and raw bacon	5 to 7 days	1 to 2 months
	Sausage made from raw chicken, turkey, pork, beef	1 to 2 days	1 to 2 months
GROUND MEATS: BEEF, POULTRY, OTHERS	Fresh ground beef, turkey, chicken, veal, pork, lamb	1 to 2 days	3 to 4 months

Category	Food Specifics	Refrigerator (40°F or below)	Freezer (0°F or below)*
WHOLE CUTS OF BEEF, VEAL, LAMB, PORK	Fresh steaks, chops, roasts	3 to 5 days	4 to 6 months
FRESH POULTRY	Chicken or turkey	1 to 2 days	9 months
SOUPS AND STEWS	Vegetable or meat added	3 to 4 days	2 to 3 months
COOKED, PREMADE MEALS	Prepped meals and casseroles	5 days	2 to 3 months

Freezer guidelines are for quality. Food kept below 0 degrees can be stored longer safely, but quality may decline.

PUTTING IT ALL INTO PRACTICE

Meal prep takes time, but it's time well spent. A few hours of work will create fuel that eases the stress of your busy life and moves you closer to health and performance.

Starting is easy; grab some ideas from the chart on the following page.

When matching up your meals with nutrition goals, use portion sizes that fulfill your specific nutrition needs. Since eating should also be fun, keep things exciting with variations you love—saying hello to herbs, spices, marinades, and healthy toppings.

As you continue to work toward your own health goals, trust yourself to start adjusting meal planning with the knowledge you gain in the process. Try new recipes and scale portion sizes up (or down) to meet your changing goals.

GO-TO OPTIONS FOR MEAL PREP

Carb sources that are easy to prepare in bulk and then divide	Fruit and vegetable sources that require less prep and still deliver the nutrients you're looking for	Protein sources that are easy to prepare in bulk and then divide	Fat sources—added during prep or served on the side	Flavor—switch these up to take the same base (protein or carb) and create an entirely different meal
Whole grain pastas and gluten-free, bean/legume-based options—all shapes and sizes	Fresh apple slices, fresh veggie sticks, baby carrots, fruit salad	Poultry: boneless, skinless breast, drumsticks, ground lean chicken and turkey	Avocado and avocado oil	Tomato-based marinara sauce
Brown rice	Frozen steamable blends	Pork: loin and tenderloin	Mixed nuts	Salsa, pico de gallo, picante
Lentils	Veggie spiralized noodles	Fish: salmon and other firm fish fillets	Cheese	Soy sauce, miso, wasabi
Mashed, baked, or sliced (sweet) potatoes	Frozen fruit for smoothies and quick-thaw for cereal and yogurt toppings	Eggs: hard-boiled, scrambled, baked in muffin cups	Bacon or pancetta, chopped	Spices and seasoning blends: Trader Joe's Everything but the Bagel Sesame Seasoning Blend, McCormick Grill Mates
Ancient grains: quinoa, sorghum, spelt, amaranth	Bags of spinach, kale, arugula, etc.	Meatballs: turkey, chicken, or lean pork from fresh or frozen meat	Coconut oil, butter, olive oil	Splash of citrus juice or grated peel
Whole grain tortillas	Steam-ready, stir-fry-ready fresh veggie blends	Soy: firm tofu cubed, seasoned, cooked	Simple homemade salad dressings	Fresh herbs—stored intact and chopped, torn, or diced before enjoying

PART 3

THIS GIRL IS ON FIRE

THE HIGH SCHOOL AND COLLEGE YEARS

As is true of many who survived high school but didn't necessarily thrive, I wouldn't go back there even for a million dollars. Conversely, I'd pay a million dollars to relive the newfound freedom and excitement of college, even though that period too had its challenging moments.

The process of navigating the last years of school carries with it a mix of stress and excitement. During these formative adult years, you'll undergo countless physical changes accompanying puberty, natural changes that are part of the transition from adolescent to adult. Fully understanding and then accepting the changes that take place during the transition to adulthood is not easy.

Moving from the comforts of home, where food is most often prepared and provided by someone else, into the world, where it's necessary to forage for your own fuel (even if this just involves taking a short walk to the dining hall) can throw some athletes into a tailspin.

When asked to reflect on their journey, some athletes mention discovering all-you-can-eat dining halls, learning to fend for and fuel themselves, fearing the Freshman 15, and learning that the diet and lifestyle of an athlete needs to be different from that of a typical student. Many reported countless missteps and life lessons, including struggles with mental health issues, and in the best of times, coming up with new coping mechanisms and overcoming obstacles, but not necessarily before graduation.

Significant physiological changes accompany the high school and college years. Many of these changes require plentiful energy to occur, and the combination of intensive training plus insufficient caloric intake can interfere with progress and growth.

Change Is in the Air: What to Expect as You Transition from Teen to Woman

▸ Increases in height: During this period, critical bone mass is laid down and protective, essential adipose tissue accumulates. Fuel this growth with adequate energy and bone-supporting micronutrients.

▸ Modifications of gait and stride: The angle from hip to knee is altered, resulting in changes in gait, stride, and landing patterns. The late teenage years carry the highest risk of knee and ACL injury: female athletes from fourteen to nineteen are among those who have the highest incidence of ACL injury. Work to adapt to changes in movement and coordination, and strength-train to fight imbalances.

▸ Increases in weight: Deposition of bone and increases in adipose tissue and muscle mass will naturally drive up the number on the scale. As for the fabled Freshman 15, don't waste time worrying about it. Instead, keep moving and building a better plate; skip late-night snacking and binge drinking and you'll easily crush this mythical foe.

▸ Changes in hormones: The rise and fall of the levels of estrogen and progesterone prior to your period and throughout each cycle result in significant mood changes and other symptoms—sometimes mild, sometimes leading you to spend the day in bed. Fight back with adequate fluids, micronutrient supplementation, and a baby aspirin if your doc approves.

▸ Fatigue: The energy required to fuel growth, increased training load, and a packed schedule is no joke. Don't skimp on sleep and don't forget to keep gas in the tank.

This is a phase in life where you effectively transition from childhood to womanhood. Even though puberty may be delayed, pubertal changes will take place and likely in full;

> **Pro Tip:** *You can't outwit mother nature. Young athletes wanting to delay puberty and the physical changes that accompany maturation have sometimes purposefully (sometimes accidentally) coupled training with inadequate food intake, slowing down the transition from youth to adult. Intensive training and negative energy balance change the hypothalamic pituitary set point at puberty, prolong the prepubertal stage, and delay the onset of menstruation, and these effects have been seen across a variety of sports. But these effects come with a terrible cost. Long-term damage and missed growth potential accompany chronic fuel deficit. Try as you might, you can't avoid the inevitable. And for better outcomes, you really don't want to. So work with your body, not against it.*

research suggests it is shifted to a later age, following bone maturation rather than chronological age. But some side effects may be permanent; catch-up growth might occur in full, but there's a better chance you'll fall short of reaching your full growth potential.

SEEK SLEEP

Chasing a dream isn't possible if you don't make time for sleep. Late nights with friends and early morning practices or classes make prioritizing sleep across high school and college years easier said than done. Training plus growth plus late nights do not equal optimal health. Still, many high school and college students fall short on this critical factor.

So why is it that nine in ten Americans prioritize just about any other aspect of daily living—sweat sessions, work, social life, and hobbies—over precious sleep? The value of sleep can't be overstated, and inadequate sleep leads to poor health, poor performance, premature fatigue, and even increased cravings and hunger.

Later on in life, inadequate sleep can even impact women's weight. Data from the Nurses' Health Study, a huge longitudinal study including over 68,000 registered nurses, found that the subjects who reported sleeping less gained more weight than those who reported sleeping more. In fact, getting just one additional hour of sleep per night had a significant impact. Over the course of the study, women who slept five hours or less a night gained 2.5 pounds more than did those who slept seven hours, while women who slept six hours a night gained 1.5 pounds more. As these associations were not affected by the amount of time participants spent exercising or the calories they consumed, it's likely that shorter duration of sleep alone can impact the rate of weight gain.

If you're tracking sleep—easy to do via your smart watch or an app—and realize that you routinely accrue fewer than eight hours, it's time to get serious about your bedtime ritual. Start implementing these strategies for better sleep.

Strategies for Sounder Sleep

Prioritize. Just as you would set aside time for a class, game, or study, set aside time for sleep. Make it habitual, starting your wind-down ritual at the same time each day. More activity calls for more rest and recovery.

Less sleep can lead to less leptin (a hormone that signals satiety) and increased ghrelin (a gut peptide associated with the sensation of hunger). So you'll be cranky as well as hungry, but your fatigue will lead you to crave high-calorie, higher-sugar choices, possibly derailing health or body composition goals you've been pursuing. You can't undo last night's late night, but you can go into a tired day knowing that you're at risk for indulging.

Skip that caffeinated cocktail. Caffeine and alcohol can totally ruin a good night's sleep. Cut out caffeine after one P.M. The more sensitive you are to the effects of caffeine, the earlier you should shut it down. Alcohol may make you sleepy, but the quality of your sleep will be poor, and you will experience a lethargic and dehydrated morning the next day. Opt instead for a relaxing beverage like chamomile tea or casein-rich warm milk. American long-distance runner Allie Ostrander relies on supplements that contain melatonin, magnesium, L-theanine, and other botanicals, but you'll want to check in with your team dietitian before you add in any supplements.

Turn off your devices. I know this is easier said than done, but the content can be stressful and the blue light is harmful. If you need to unwind, check out something other than the nightly news or your social media feed. Instead, grab a relaxing magazine or a novel. Still not sleepy? Grab a textbook. Chances are you'll be asleep in no time.

Create a restful environment. Cool, dark, and quiet are your friends. If your roommate and you are on different schedules, invest in a sleeping mask and earplugs or noise-canceling headphones to create a spa-like environment.

COLLEGIATE AND HIGH SCHOOL PRO TIPS: LEAN ON *THE LIGHT* FROM OTHERS

You're not the first one to navigate this sometimes awkward phase of life, and you won't be the last. To help you on your way, here are some tips and experiences shared by those lighting the path before you.

Pro Tips from Stephanie Bruce

Describing her relationship with food as a young athlete, Stephanie Bruce says there really wasn't one. There was never talk about the impact a food might have on performance or weight, perhaps because Bruce grew up with brothers, and men and women address the topic of food in a strikingly different fashion. "We simply didn't talk about bodies and food. We ate a mix of all foods. There wasn't a stigma that differentiated boys and girls. And so there were no gender-based barriers in our house. Food was fuel and nourishment." Embrace Bruce's body positivity and food neutrality by shifting your mindset. Remember that food is made to nourish us. Her nutrition foundation is strong because she was taught early on that food needn't be correlated with weight, nor was weight necessarily correlated with running performance.

Bruce adds: "I gained fifteen pounds of 'comfort foods' across my early college days."

Bruce sought solace in food but found that this weight hampered her performance when running, simply because her body wasn't built to carry comfort foods. As her mileage went up, her body faltered under the stress and responded with stress fractures. So she did some research about how to eat better and realized that collegiate athletes simply must fuel differently, and late-night pizza wasn't the best option.

"When my nutrition undulates, it's due to still working to determine intolerances or which foods work to fuel and which ones definitely don't. Early college years taught me that low energy plus high mileage spelled disaster. Self-taught, I dove into nutrition to determine the right energy levels for me. I later cofounded Picky Bars to supply clean and simple fuel to athletes like me who were looking for simple fuel that was nutrient dense and supported recovery with the right mix of protein and carbs. I learned to consciously add more fuel as my mileage increased."

Pro Tips from Allie Ostrander

After seeing older athletes mature and then slow down, Allie Ostrander was determined to fight mother nature. With a fear of losing control and losing performance, she began restricting across her preteen years, effectively suppressing puberty but at a high cost. Rather than viewing the transition to womanhood as gaining size, strength, and power, Allie saw it as a death sentence to speed. But this suppression of puberty eventually catches up to young women, resulting in poor bone health, low energy levels, an inability to recover, and an inability to gain strength. After seeking therapy and battling to return to the sport she loves, Allie worries about the damage she's done. "Our body has a level where we feel and perform our best, but we unnaturally chase some number [on the scale]. Now I listen to my body. It reminds me if I'm not fueling well."

DEAR YOUNGER, HUNGRY ME: ALLIE OSTRANDER

Can you be from Alaska without exhibiting toughness and grit? After meeting Allie and hearing how's she's navigated the twists and turns of running and life, you'll realize she is as tough as they come. As a specialist in the steeplechase, Allie is a three-time NCAA champion, with thirteen all-American honors, despite experiencing injury, setbacks, and mental health challenges. She shows all of us what is possible when you speak up, seek help, and prioritize your health; you keep coming back and crushing it. Allie coaches at Seattle Pacific University, dedicates time to support future superstars and advocate for mental health, isn't afraid to call out the critics who promote negative body-image talk across women's sports, and selflessly, transparently shares her own journey to light the way for others.

Dear Younger Allie,

I would say that you are hungrier too, but I think if I'm honest, I'm just as hungry now as I have ever been. I don't just mean hungry in a stomach-growling, "dreaming of a juicy burger" way, either. I also mean it in the "driven to do whatever it takes to be successful" way. I'm hungrier than ever for the pursuit of my athletic and nonathletic goals, and a big reason for that is I've learned that hunger is not the enemy.

There will be people who tell you not to grab seconds because then you "won't run as fast next year." There will be reporters who attribute your success purely to your small stature. There will be doctors who tell you not to worry about a missing period or a low body weight because "you have a runner's body." It is important—imperative—for you to realize that those people are wrong. While they focus on the body that carries you, they can't see the brain that ignores the burn in your legs and pushes through regardless of how hard it gets. They can't comprehend the cost of the brutal training sessions you put in week after week as you fight to beat the boys in practice every day. They don't understand the genetic components of fitness and athleticism that have no impact on physical appearance. Be careful what—if anything—you take away from their advice. They see only the surface of you, and it is the contents that truly make you incredible.

You will spend years focused on the surface of yourself, thinking that manipulating this will make you successful. You will start to see hunger as the enemy. Something to be ignored, squashed, and avoided at all costs. The primary focus of training will become changing the way you look instead of the way you feel. Food won't be used to fuel training and reap the maximum benefits because, over the years, food has become feared. It is seen as a training eraser that will only hold you back from being your best. This fear will drive you to train hard and pursue your athletic goals, but it will do so with total disregard for your health or happiness. While you may see success, it will come with a side of isolation, sadness, and most of all, injury.

It will take a while for you to realize that these effects aren't a coincidence. They won't go away with time, only morph and change and trick you again and again into thinking that your outward appearance determines your success. Your hunger for fuel will continually grow, but your insistence on ignoring it will increase at an equal level. Eventually, your desire and obsession with ignoring hunger and fearing food will take up so much space in your brain that there will be less room for the pursuit of your athletic and nonathletic goals. These will get pushed to the back and ignored, even though they were supposed to be the reason for wanting a certain body.

Finally, after years of injuries and heartbreak, you will realize that avoiding hunger hasn't made you a better runner or person. It has only stripped you of your happiness, health, and ability to train consistently. It won't be easy, but you will begin to shed the belief that your appearance determines your ability. You will learn to honor your hunger and fuel your training so you can recover and benefit from those difficult sessions. Slowly, as you finally feed your physical hunger, the hunger for your goals will return. Instead of dedicating all your brain space to ignoring hunger, you treat hunger as what it is—a signal that your body needs food—and move on with your day, allowing that space in your brain to be taken up by far more important things. Hunger for running a new PR. Hunger for building the running community. Hunger for raising awareness of eating disorders. Hunger for time spent laughing with family and friends. Because the best type of hunger is the one that growls for you to live a full and happy life.

Sincerely,
Allie O

You see, the transition from child to adolescent to adult is peppered with discovery and achievement, but it's not without stress, turmoil, and dark days. And women are likely to have more than their fair share of dark days. During childhood, boys and girls have comparable rates of depression; in adulthood, women account for the majority of clinical cases of depression. This struggle emerges as early as age thirteen to fourteen, which roughly corresponds to the midpoint of pubertal development, and the hormonal flux that occurs as a result of it. Researchers are still uncovering the system(s) responsible for the incidence of depression, but if you too are feeling lower than you think is right or "normal" or optimal, speak up. You can't fight an invisible cloak of darkness by yourself. Furthermore, you don't have to. Ask for help as soon as possible so you can start to build a foundation of coping skills, positive thinking, belief in self, and unshakable mental health.

Pro Tip from Molly Seidel

Don't be so hard on yourself. When asked what she would have done differently during collegiate years, without pause Molly Seidel said she would have been kinder to her younger self. You'll find this wisdom echoed in many Dear Younger, Hungry Me letters.

Pro Tips from Tatyana McFadden

When Tatyana was asked her perspective on food, inclusivity, and body positivity among young athletes, she said that she finds it encouraging that conversations are finally happening. "I do think that we are moving in the right direction with athletes at the college level and above. What we do not see is conversation among high school athletes, let alone youth with disabilities . . . When I was in high school I had to learn to accept that I was built differently. And that my strong arms were a gift. On my high school track team, we did not have conversations about recovery and what to eat after workouts." If your team isn't having these conversations, either, you're now equipped with the knowledge to start them. Tatyana goes on: "When my career as an elite athlete began in 2004, direction regarding nutrition from Team USA was limited, but that has changed dramatically. Nutrition for athletes with disabilities is now tracked and studied, and all athletes have a regular check-in with the nutritionist." But more work needs to be done. The focus on nutrition needs to be continuous, more data needs to be collected, and the information needs to be accessible to all.

DEAR YOUNGER, HUNGRY ME: TATYANA McFADDEN

Life is a process of embracing the gifts you've been given and building upon them. With her gifts, Tatyana has built an inspirational legacy. She was born in Russia with spina bifida and paralyzed from the waist down. She spent the first six years of her life without the aid of a wheelchair and relied on her willpower and her own two arms to get about. She embodied *yo sama*, Russian for "I can do it myself." She recalls, "I knew that if I wanted to play with the other children, no one was going to help me join them. It was up to me to move." At age six, she was adopted and moved to the United States, where she was introduced to just about every sport imaginable and excelled in just about all of them. Her athletic accomplishments include twenty Paralympic medals (eight gold, eight silver, and four bronze medals won between 2004 and Tokyo, and a prized Olympic medal won in her birth country, for Nordic skiing), and twenty-four major marathon titles. She is continuously breaking down barriers to access and working to promote capabilities in sport. Tatyana reminds us that "life isn't about what you don't have. It's what you do with the gifts you are given." When faced with adversity, she's overcome it again and again. She's never stopped to question if something is possible. She's been a vocal advocate for equality across sport and life. I'm honored to share her letter and story.

Dear Younger, Hungry Tatyana,

I want to tell you how incredibly proud I am of you and how far you have come. I know that life has not been easy, but you are doing everything you can to find your path and use the wonderful gifts that you have been given. Who could have known that your first six years in an orphanage would play a role in making you the athlete you would become? Food was scarce as you ate mostly beets, cabbage, and potatoes—who knew that today these would be considered the ultimate "power foods"! Or that walking on your hands would build the strength in your upper body that would propel you to victory in the future? You had nothing, but you made it seem like you had the world.

Coming to the United States will bring lots of firsts. Doctor visits, school, and trying lots of different food. When you first try ice cream, you may think it is too cold . . . and ask your parents to put it in the microwave because you do not understand that it is supposed to be cold! You will learn that meals are partly about "food" but also about gathering as a family to talk about the day. You will learn that "family" is a lot more than parents as you meet your grandma, who will cook most of your meals. You may start out as a picky eater, but soon you will learn to enjoy food and to try new things. As you get older, you will look back and realize that you not only love food, but you love learning about how the proper foods can build body strength.

High school will be an awkward time as you start to understand your body and work to "fit in." The differences in your body will become real to you. You will face discrimination, but it will not stop you—it will only make you stronger. Your decision to pursue sports will be the most pivotal decision of your high school years. In some ways, it will save your life. It will build your self-confidence and make you strong. You will win your first international races and begin to see your future as an athlete and an advocate.

As you explore your racing career, you will need to learn more about the importance of training and nutrition. You will attend a camp in Georgia which will be a turning point. There you will learn that you need to change your eating habits if you want to get stronger, better, and faster. Good carbs, more protein, healthy fats will be the answer. When you make these changes, you will find that they will make a huge difference in your performance.

College will be a wonderful adventure! You will love learning—and love participating in not one, but two sports. You will experience ups and downs (as all college students do) but will find support from your loving family. You will learn that adapting to change is a challenge—but it is also an adventure. During these years you will try running marathons . . . and it will change your life. With the addition of endurance events, you will learn even more about the critical role that proper nutrition and mental preparation play in success.

As you get older and approach your thirties, please remember that your body is always changing—and you will need to change along with it. You must take more time to recover, and really focus on foods that help you to recover easily. You should celebrate all your victories—and learn from the races where you don't come in first. Remember that life is a marathon, not a sprint. Be kind to yourself and others . . . don't forget to find the fun in between the work . . . and I know you will live an immensely happy life.

Love,
Tatyana!

CAMPUS 101:
STAYING FUELED WHEN YOU'RE ON YOUR OWN

DINING HALL: BUILDING THE BEST PLATE

T
alk about reinventing yourself! Nothing has changed quite as significantly as the menus in college dining halls. Sit-down service, weekly rotating menus of comfort food, and boring buffets offering mystery meats and potatoes are far less common. Modern dining halls are more often à la carte, with options ranging from taco bars to salad bars to build-your-own pizza/smoothie/wrap/omelet/sushi/you name it. Today's dining halls offer a veritable smorgasbord, with an endless variety of flavors, forms, and textures. And just about everything can be customized to meet your nutrient needs, allergen concerns, and taste preferences. But the options can be downright dizzying. What *should* you, as a collegiate athlete, choose?

What should your plate look like when meal prep is impossible, there's no kitchen in your dorm room, and you're responsible for procuring meals and snacks that fuel and sustain? Herein lie the perks of the dining hall—access to readily prepared meals (no cooking required!) and an endless array of healthy and delicious options.

Whether you're a D1 athlete on scholarship, a D3 athlete balancing a love of your sport with academics, a club player, or an intramural champ, prioritizing nutrition and designing

> **Pro Tip:** Today's collegiate dining halls offer something for everyone, with accommodations made for food allergies, religious and ethnic preferences, and other dietary needs. Swing by and find the dining hall manager or lead staff and have an open conversation about the specialized fuel you require for health and other reasons. They are there to help you! Building rapport will also build your confidence in knowing there's fuel available to support you, and this quick stop will save you time and energy in the long run.

a plate that works for *you* is often the difference between optimal performance and injury, setbacks, and a slow decline.

THE ATHLETE'S PLATE

The plate of an athlete looks different from the plate of other college-age students because the demands placed on an athlete's body and schedule are different. Luckily, the modern dining hall offers countless options, which can be exciting and can definitely be overwhelming.

> **Pro Tip:** Division I and II NCAA student-athletes can receive unlimited meals and snacks in conjunction with their athletics participation. With the goal of meeting the nutritional needs of all student-athletes, this provision is in addition to the meal plan provided as part of a full scholarship. Prior to this change, scholarship student-athletes received three meals a day or a food stipend. D3 students may be provided meals and snacks on game day and snacks following workouts, practices, and games, even outside of that sport's season.

Here are some tips from collegiate superstars and sports dietitians to help you develop a winning plan for the campus cafeteria.

YOU'RE ON YOUR OWN: Entering the adult world of total food freedom can be stressful, especially for athletes. There's no one to look over your shoulder and remind you to refuel and recover, and *you* are now responsible for setting aside time to restock and replenish your larder. There's also no one to ask if you've finished your green beans before you grab dessert or to give you the side-eye when you choose pizza for the eighth dinner in a row. The freedom can be both liberating and terrifying. Remember: just because you've left the nest doesn't mean nutrition is no-holds-barred. Choices and portions matter. Nutrient timing and adequate fueling are paramount. Your bites build a better you, so make them count.

OWN YOUR PLATE: The foods you choose set the foundation for your energy levels, your muscle recovery, and the prevention of injury. Forget the idea that there are "good" and "bad" foods, but be aware that your choices do have an impact on both your athletic and your academic performance. "This really isn't about the perception of 'eating good,'" says EXOS sports dietitian Amanda Carlson-Phillips. "Many of us are sensitive about what's on our plate and [have a] perception or feeling of being judged. I love to see athletes flip the switch and view food and nutrition as not just checking a box or achieving a number on the scale or specific body composition, but to truly unlock their potential peak performance."

CHOOSE YOUR OWN ADVENTURE: In the dining hall, the world is literally your buffet. It's packed with enticing items that can move you toward (and away from) your goals. The setting may look different, but your nutrition goals should remain the same: load up on colorful, nutrient-packed whole foods, and go light on empty calories and processed junk. While every bite matters, one meal or one food choice won't make or break you. It's the cumulative choices you make over time that will drive you in one direction or another. So if you find yourself sitting down to a comfort meal or an everything-fried Friday special, that's perfectly okay. Eat across a spectrum of *sometimes* and *always* foods rather than employing an all-or-nothing approach.

PLAN FOR SUCCESS: Poor planning equals poor implementation equals minimized results, Carlson-Phillips advises, adding: "Setting up the right process to ensure that you have access to great food choices is key to performance and even lifelong health. It doesn't matter whether you're making your meal, eating out, or having it delivered. What matters is knowing what your body needs and ensuring you have access to it. If you consider your nutrition and fueling strategy [as equivalent to] your cardiovascular and strength training and other aspects of your approach to sport, then you'll win, and that victory will translate to the field, track, course, and court."

TIME IT RIGHT: Finding the time to procure and consume adequate optimal nutrition is a common obstacle facing collegiate athletes and newly minted adults. As you run from class to practice or from work to the gym, finding time to fuel can be *hard*. Your schedule and commitments will change from day to day, but the critical and science-based need for pre-fueling, replenishment, and recovery will never waver. Instead of falling victim to underfueling because of overscheduling, aim for small meals and snacks to keep energy levels steady and avoid the two- to four-hour digestion window needed to settle larger meals. If you're within an hour or two of your sweat sesh and need a pick-me-up, focus on optimal hydration (water plus electrolytes) and easy-to-digest carbs with a small amount of protein and fat, such as a bagel with nut butter and sliced fruit. After your workout or practice, rehydrate on your way to the dining hall and eat some high-quality protein within thirty to sixty minutes. Learn more about nutrient timing on page 176.

STOP THE SWIRL: You might feel paralyzed by anxiety before you even set foot on campus, let alone enter the dining hall. Take a deep breath. Remember that when it's done right, optimal collegiate fueling can and will meet the demands that the sport makes on your body and health. But if you're chasing some arbitrary number on the scale or living in fear of the Freshman 15 and cut back rather than fuel yourself properly, you are bound to break. The Freshman 15 is more myth than truth. It has more to do with your social life and drinking than it does with what you choose in the dining hall.

Fear of weight gain, stress over the newness of it all, and packed schedules can send any co-ed running for comfort, let alone a collegiate athlete who has been recruited to deliver a high level of excellence.

Pro Tip: Allie Ostrander described the transition from high school to college as being "stressful in an exciting way." She added that when you are equipped with a meal plan and access to dining halls and training tables, it can be easy to find fast fuel to rehydrate and recover. But if your schedule is packed, it's also easy not to eat enough. The threat of the Freshman 15 looms large, sparking fears of overfueling and confusion about what to choose. Allie wasn't the only one to turn to food restriction as a way to both cope with and quiet her fears. "I always believed I could be a better runner if I was smaller. I know now that's not the case, and I regret the long-term damage I've likely done."

NORMAL RULES DON'T APPLY: The schedule of a collegiate athlete is demanding, and what's on your plate needs to stand up to the grueling task of supporting full-time performance, academics, and the rest of life. Often, normal rules about how to eat don't apply when you're working tirelessly to fuel both athletic and educational performance as well as health. Stephanie Bruce realized this during her first year of collegiate competition. She joined her friends for late-night pizza and learned the hard way that this type of fuel wasn't right for high performance. An uptick in weight coupled with a demanding schedule of increasing mileage resulted in a stress fracture. Bruce took a step back, realized she'd need to sacrifice some late-night socials if performance was a priority, and acknowledged that her plate simply couldn't look the same as her classmates. She researched the types of fuel that might spark her to be faster and stronger, confidently built an elite athlete's plate, and never looked back.

PRIORITIZE GOOD NUTRITION: When it comes down to healthy eating, you must prioritize making good nutrition happen consistently. Day in and day out, choose to make choices that move you in the right direction. That means building a plate packed with foods rich in macro- and micronutrients—fruits, vegetables, whole grains, lean proteins, and dairy—and containing fewer of the foods commonly ordered in a fast-food drive-through. Don't skip meals; do keep energy levels high by intentionally snacking between meals, and mindfully eat adequate food at mealtimes.

BE SPORT SPECIFIC: Dietitian and former collegiate runner Sarah Sharp says: "There are simple strategies to keep in mind when navigating the dining hall. When you build your plate, the demands of your sport should factor in your choices. If you're a distance runner, it is easy to gravitate toward carbs after practice, because your glycogen [energy] stores are running low and your body craves to refuel that energy. However, protein is also key for recovery and building/maintaining lean muscle, and your body needs fat to boost your energy intake, to absorb nutrients, and to support your health. Endurance athletes should aim to make at least half the plate carbs, a fourth of the plate protein, and a fourth of the plate fruit and veggies. Team and strength athletes need more protein to support muscle and strength, so build a plate with a third carbs, a third protein, and a third fiber-rich color."

YOU DO YOU: The dining hall and training tables are the easiest place to get caught up in keeping up with the Joneses. But your plate does not need to mirror that of teammates. One size does not fit all. The demands of sport and your unique physiology mean you need a more personalized plate.

"It was frustrating (annoying?) to see other athletes underfuel and even make temporary improvements while I was eating to fuel my running and answer hunger and appetite," said Boston Marathon winner Des Linden. But rather than fall into restriction and the fatigue and injury concomitant with it, Linden chose to chart her own course. "I just said, 'You know what, you go ahead and underfuel. I'll keep eating and getting stronger, and by the end of the season, you'll break down and I'll kick your ass in competition.'" By eating wisely, she was able to fuel the grind successfully.

WATCH YOUR PORTIONS, PLEASE: All-you-can-eat dining halls can be to your benefit, or not. It can be tempting to load plate after plate, effectively "getting your money's worth," but this investment pays off only if you're pursuing more mass and weight gain. After all, there's a good chance that someday your levels of physical activity will decline and your metabolism will too. Whatever your performance and weight goals may be, listening to your body and respecting hunger signals remains paramount.

"If you can, grab a snack—a granola bar or a piece of whole fruit to take with you—so you'll have a solution should your energy levels start to dip," recommends Sharp. Remember, make that second course count—continue to choose nutrient-dense choices that build your energy reserves, support your recovery, and prime your tank for the next workout. Need ideas? Check out the tips below.

DINING HALL PICKS

Food Group	Food Item
PROTEIN	Grilled, roasted, or baked chicken breast, pork loin and tenderloin, beef (trimmed or lean, ground), baked fish, legumes and lentils, nut butters, vegan meat-replacement/plant-based meat substitutes
GRAINS	Rice, pasta, quinoa, corn, baked potato and sweet potato, cereals Whole grain bread, rolls, wraps, tortillas
VEGGIES	Steamed, blanched, or sautéed broccoli, carrots, cauliflower, squash, beets Entrée salads with protein, grain toppers, and plant-based oils and fats can make a great meal; make sure yours include adequate calories and choose these outside of training hours to avoid high fiber.

DINING HALL PICKS

Food Group	Food Item
FRUIT	Whole fruits (apple, banana, orange); fruit salad with berries, melon; fruit puree pouches and applesauce
DAIRY/DAIRY ALTERNATIVES	Milk, chocolate milk, fortified soy milk, fortified nut milks (typically high in calcium but not protein), Greek yogurt, cheese
HYDRATION FOODS/BEVERAGES	Water, sports drinks, smoothies, soup (great way to get extra protein, veggies, and sodium)

OFF-CAMPUS 101

You've moved from the dining hall to off-campus housing, and now you're responsible for both procuring and preparing your food. Fantastic. No, seriously—this period of life that may feel like a heavy lift is a perfect time to perfect your cooking skills and ability to plan meals, as well as learn how to budget.

Remember that while performance nutrition can get complex, the foundation remains simple: variety, nutrient density, and adequacy. Tatyana McFadden recalls working to eat healthy on a budget, noting that with careful planning, you can check both boxes. Grab canned, frozen, and bulk items, opting to make simple meals at home from scratch rather than buying pricier semi-prepared processed meals. McFadden adds that eating healthy doesn't have to be overly fancy, "clean," or gourmet. Resist falling into the mindset that in order to perform, you must ensure that everything you eat has to be expensive or organic. There's no science to support such ideas, there's no need to break the bank when eating healthfully, and I can assure you that pristine and pricy plates won't guarantee you a place on the podium.

Healthy eating can be achieved on any budget. Just keep the following tips in mind prior to hitting the grocery store:

1. **Make a grocery list and stick with it.** Plan your meals and snacks ahead of time to assure a stock of adequate fuel so you'll have available what your body *needs* but save dollars as you skip what your taste buds might *want*.

2. **Never shop on an empty stomach.** This number one rule of frugal shoppers will prevent you from making impulse buys and coming home with tons of overly processed and pricy junk food.

3. **Shop seasonally and on sale.** Fresh fruits and vegetables taste better, are more nutrient dense, and are less expensive when bought in season.

Pro Tip: *Stock up, prep, and then freeze for future smoothie making or to thaw and enjoy when winter hits.*

4. **Incorporate canned, dried, and frozen.** Leslie Bonci, a venerated sports dietitian and consultant to individual athletes and professional teams, recommends economical and high-quality canned, dried, and frozen fruits, veggies, beans, and lentils. These items are nutrient dense, are usually less expensive than fresh, and have a shelf life that allows for stocking up. Choose fruits packed in 100 percent juice (not syrup) and choose canned vegetables with no added salt and plain frozen veggies. (Add your own salt, seasoning, and sauce as needed.)

5. **Stick with the essentials.** You don't need fancy gadgets or appliances to bring healthy eating to life. Equip your off-campus canteen with some decent cutlery, a pot in which to cook pasta, rice, and oats, and a skillet for stir-frying veggies and tofu, and round out your equipment with a sheet pan/baking sheet on which to roast chicken and sliced veggies or to prepare other one-sheet meals.

6. **Build on the familiar.** Start with low-maintenance inexpensive favorites like mac and cheese, ramen, or canned soup and add extra nutrition with a bag of frozen broccoli or vegetable medley, grilled chicken strips, chopped fresh vegetables, canned beans, and more. While the base of the entrée may be inexpensive, the meal will lean more gourmet, and the simple additions will add color and nutrients to your dish.

7. **Buy in bulk.** Why spend extra on individual microwave-ready potatoes, single-serve packets of instant oatmeal, or ready-to-eat cups of macaroni when you can buy pounds of the main ingredient for pennies on the dollar? Bonci suggests that rather than break the bank, you stock up on pantry essentials like russet potatoes, grains, and lentils, invest time prepping (see page 103 for meal prep help), and package up and refrigerate servings for the week ahead or freeze and then quickly defrost them when timing is tight and you're ravenous post-workout.

ADVENTURE AWAITS: FUEL FOR THE ROAD TRIP

What do you do when your schedule calls for an away game, match, or race? Eating on the road can be challenging, especially when you don't know where you'll be having your pre-competition dinner or whether you'll need to fill your backpack with snacks.

Meals and snacks matter, as both fuel your muscles and your mental focus when you step onto the course or playing field. Ideally, you'll be handed a bento box that the team sports dietitian has carefully put together to deliver balanced energy and hydration. But more often the coach may pack supplies to make simple sandwiches or hand you a few bucks to forage for food wherever the bus may stop. In this situation, it's best to take matters into your own hands. The way you fuel on the way to the competition and while you're there will have a big impact on your energy during your event and after it.

SNACK EARLY AND OFTEN. Keep your energy levels steady with a small supply of fuel across the day. Experiment to find something that sits well on your stomach. If the staff or coach also supplies your favorite, great. If not, bring your own.

SHOW UP HYDRATED. The average athlete shows up to a workout and then a competition in a dehydrated state, which negatively affects performance. Don't be average. Sip on fluids throughout your travels (water is best, but sports drinks can help top off your energy and electrolytes) and maintain your fluid intake so your urine remains light yellow in color. (For more tips on hydration, see page 202).

STAY FUELED. Multiple bouts of competition during the day, or travel back and forth to the team hotel, can make it difficult to stay fueled. Avoid hitting empty with small meals and snacks, consistent hydration, and a recovery snack (150 to 300 calories, including 15 to 30 grams of protein and 30 or more grams of carbohydrate) to enjoy within 30 minutes of the time your competition ends.

SKIP THE HEAVY STUFF. High-fat, fast casual fare is not your friend when it comes to fueling your body before and between games. Spoiler alert: I've tried such foods pre-game and we didn't win. Large portions of food full of fats and carbohydrates create digestive havoc, demanding significant blood flow for digestion, insulin secretion for blood glucose absorption, and more. Better options for a road trip include light, small portions of pasta or rice bowls, sub sandwiches, grilled chicken wraps, and entrée salads, as long as fiber doesn't upset your stomach.

Need more ideas on how to pack your travel snack supplies? Follow these tips from Sarah Sharp.

1. **Don't try new things on race/game day.** Practice days are the perfect time to see which foods agree with you if you eat within an hour or two of training. Explore options until you find which foods energize you. Use practice days to map out food choices for race day.

2. **Focus on easy-to-digest carbohydrates prior to competition.** Avoid spicy foods and foods full of fat, protein, and fiber before your event. Simple carbohydrates are a quick source of energy that are gentle on the stomach and support muscle function.

3. **Protein and carbs are the best duo for travel days and recovery after competition.** Whether you're sitting in a travel van or on a bus, driving for hours on the road probably means a long time between meals. Snacking is a must to help your muscles recover and to begin refueling your body's energy stores. Pair a carb and a protein snack to keep your body well fueled. Healthy fats are also a bonus to help your body stave off inflammation.

4. **Salty foods and electrolyte drinks help with hydration.** You can't avoid a good sweat when you're giving 100 percent effort. And under hot or humid conditions, the sweat factor will only increase, depleting your body of critical fluid volume and essential electrolytes. Post-competition, grab a bag of pretzels or an alternate salty snack, a water bottle, and a sports drink to help replace what's lost.

5. **Strategize your snack times.** Try an easy-to-digest carb source like a banana, a granola bar, or applesauce when competing within an hour. Hungry after dinner? Top off the tank before bed with a balanced snack offering fat, protein, and complex carbs (your blood glucose will thank you later).

TRAVEL TIPS: FOODS AND SNACKS TO PACK

Carbs	Fruit: oranges, apples, bananas, peaches, applesauce, dried fruit, fruit and vegetable pouches Easy-to-digest carbs: bananas, animal crackers, applesauce, granola bars, fruit snacks, English muffins, dried fruit, fig bars, bagels, pita chips Whole grains: popcorn, whole grain bread/crackers, instant oatmeal
Protein	Nut butters and nuts, beef jerky, tuna packets, cheese sticks, Greek yogurt, hard-boiled eggs, whey or plant-based protein shakes

TRAVEL TIPS: FOODS AND SNACKS TO PACK

Carb + Protein Combos	Peanut butter and jelly, high-protein energy bars, fruit and granola Greek yogurt parfait, cheese stick and crackers, turkey and cheese tortilla wrap, hummus and pita or pretzels, trail mix
Salty Snacks	Pretzels, crackers, saltines, salted nuts, olives, sunflower seeds
Fluids	Sparkling water, electrolyte-containing drinks and sports drinks, shelf-stable chocolate milk, coconut water, 100% fruit juice boxes

GAME DAY 101: FUELING UP FOR INTENSE MATCHES AND TOURNAMENTS

For start-and-stop sports, you typically have more time between games to digest and absorb fuel. Your sport demands energy from carbs and protein to support strength. Throughout the day, choose light satisfying fare (i.e., no chicken fingers and fries) that supplies carbs for energy, a hint of fat for nourishment, and a boost of protein to make you feel full and to support recovery and muscle health.

PUTTING IT INTO PRACTICE

Scenario 1: You're leaving campus early Saturday morning for a round robin, featuring a game Saturday afternoon, one Saturday evening, and one Sunday morning.

Timing	Goal	Fuel
FRIDAY NIGHT	Fully stock up glycogen stores and the amino acid pool so you'll be prepped with energy and strength, respectively, for tomorrow's matches.	Enjoy a high-carb, moderate-protein dinner complete with alcohol-free fluids (alcohol is often banned by teams; excessive alcohol dehydrates, contributes to poor sleep quality, and negatively impacts reaction time and overall performance). Fill ¼ of your plate with veggies, ¼ with lean protein, ½ with whole grain carbs (pasta, rice, ancient grains).

PUTTING IT INTO PRACTICE

Scenario 1: You're leaving campus early Saturday morning for a round robin, featuring a game Saturday afternoon, one Saturday evening, and one Sunday morning.

Timing	Goal	Fuel
SATURDAY MORNING	You've got time to digest your food, so fully top off the tank and fend off hunger.	Fill your water bottle, grab a to-go breakfast for the ride (protein shake plus dry cereal, egg sandwich, protein smoothie, or PB and banana on whole grain bread). Pack a serving of fruit for later.
SATURDAY MIDMORNING, 60 TO 90 MINUTES BEFORE THE GAME	Top off your nearly full tank with easy-to-digest fuel and fluids, assuring you've got high-octane, ready-to-burn fuel in the tank.	Water, 16-ounce sports drink, handful of animal crackers or piece of fruit.
SATURDAY POSTGAME MEAL	Proactively prep for tomorrow's game: rehydrate, refuel, recover.	Whether fast casual fare or sit-down restaurant, lean light, with a half sandwich (lean protein, lettuce, veggies, light on the mayo) and a bowl of broth-based soup or a salad topped with grilled chicken, dressing on the side, plus a whole grain roll.
SATURDAY MIDAFTERNOON, 60 TO 90 MINUTES BEFORE THE GAME	You topped off the tank at lunch, right? Grab a bite of something easy to digest and hydrate to assure you've got high-octane fuel in the tank ready when it's go-time.	Water, 16-ounce sports drink, handful of animal crackers or a piece of fruit.
SATURDAY POSTGAME MEAL	Fully stock up glycogen stores and the amino acid pool so you'll be prepped with energy and strength for tomorrow.	Moderate-high carbs, moderate protein, alcohol-free fluids. Fill ¼ of your plate with veggies, ¼ with lean protein, ½ with whole grain carbs (pasta, rice, ancient grains).
SUNDAY BREAKFAST	The closer you are to go-time, the less time you have to digest, so the lighter the meal. Grab some familiar carbs and a bit of protein to power you through the game.	Cereal and milk, fresh fruit and yogurt, bagel and nut butter, or scrambled egg on toast; 16-ounce water.
SUNDAY POSTGAME	Rehydrate with 16 to 32 ounces of water, refuel with carbohydrates, recover with 30 grams of protein.	Protein smoothie made with fruit and veggies or grilled chicken sandwich on whole grain wrap with fresh veggies.

RACE DAY 101: FUELING UP FOR EVENTS AND BACK-TO-BACK COMPETITIONS

You'll benefit from several small meals or snacks rather than heavy meals, which take longer to digest and can wreak havoc on your gastrointestinal system during competition. I recommend a light intake of fat, a moderate intake of protein, and a high intake of carbohydrate across competition days. This will keep your energy levels high and your glycogen stores stocked and primed to perform, thus leaving you less sore and fatigued after your race.

PUTTING IT INTO PRACTICE

Scenario 2: You've got a meet all day Saturday, with races peppered across the day. Your first heat is midmorning, the semis are in the afternoon, and the finals are just before six P.M. Alternatively, you could run/swim one distance in the morning, another distance 90 minutes later, and anchor the relay in the evening.

Timing	Goal	Fuel
FRIDAY NIGHT DINNER	Fully stock up glycogen stores and the amino acid pool so you'll be prepped with energy and strength, respectively, for tomorrow's matches.	Enjoy a high-carb, moderate protein dinner, without alcohol. Fill ¼ of your plate with veggies, ¼ with lean protein, ½ with whole grain carbs (pasta, rice, ancient grains). If you're still hungry, have an extra serving of carbs.
SATURDAY EARLY MORNING BREAKFAST	You've got limited time to digest, so go light and simply top off the tank.	16 to 32 ounces of water with or without electrolytes. Grab a to-go breakfast as you head to the meet: protein powder plus oats plus dried fruit, egg white on an English muffin, or PB and jam on a whole grain tortilla. Stash a granola bar and piece of fruit for later.
SATURDAY, 60 TO 90 MINUTES BEFORE THE RACE	Your tank should be full, but fend off hunger and thirst as needed.	Water, 16-ounce sports drink, handful of animal crackers if hunger strikes.
SATURDAY, 30 MINUTES AFTER THE MORNING RACE	Proactively prep for the next race: rehydrate, replace what you've lost.	Given the limited time before the next race, don't overfuel or you'll be busy digesting when you need to be racing. Grab a light half sandwich, a bowl of rehydrating broth-based soup, 16 ounces of chocolate milk, or some pretzels with hummus.

PUTTING IT INTO PRACTICE

Timing	Goal	Fuel
SATURDAY, 60 TO 90 MINUTES BEFORE THE AFTERNOON RACE	Fend off hunger and thirst as needed.	Water, 16-ounce sports drink, handful of pretzels or an energy bar if hunger strikes.
SATURDAY, 30 MINUTES AFTER THE AFTERNOON RACE	You've got a bit more time before the evening's finals but still don't have enough time to digest a large, heavy meal. Have a bite of easy-to-digest fuel and fluids.	Water, protein smoothie (whey/dairy plus fruit and veggies), savory oatmeal, or grilled chicken sandwich on whole grain wrap with fresh veggies. No heavy fare or you'll be working to digest while competing!
SATURDAY, 60 MINUTES BEFORE THE EVENING RACE	Grab some familiar carbs and a bit of protein to fend off hunger and fuel your speed.	Cereal and milk, yogurt and granola, bagel and nut butter, or scrambled egg on toast. 16-ounce water. Nervous stomach? Water plus electrolytes and an energy bar.
SATURDAY, POST-RACE MEAL	You've stocked up carbs all day. Now's the time to replace spent fluids and energy but prioritize protein and fat to facilitate recovery and nourishment.	Moderate carbs, moderate protein, moderate-fiber foods plus alcohol-free fluids (you may be celebrating, but alcohol can hamper rehydration and recovery). Fill ⅓ of your plate with veggies, ⅓ with lean protein, ⅓ with complex carbs (whole grains, sweet potatoes, lentils).

A Note About Alcohol: There's no getting around the fact that drinking is a big part of college. As difficult as it can be, it's always best to refrain. Excessive intake of alcohol dehydrates the body, contributes to poor sleep quality, and negatively impacts reaction time and overall performance. You worked so hard to earn a place on the college team, and your team and coach are relying on you. It's just not worth giving in to peer pressure and effectively sacrificing all you've worked so hard for. When the starting gun fires, you'll be glad you resisted temptation.

MOM ON THE RUN

Asked to name the hardest job on the planet, I would immediately say being a mother. Indeed, there are likely as many challenges to being a mother as there are mothers in the world. Over time these challenges rapidly appear, disappear, and sometimes reappear, reminding us that motherhood offers us little that is permanent or guaranteed.

As athletes, we're indoctrinated to believe that if we try hard enough, even the most audacious goals can become reality. But when it comes to creating life, it's not as simple as wishing, hoping, and working at it. And while society might hint that the prevalence of infertility and miscarriages, disruption in menstrual cycles, or perturbations of hormone levels are common, the topics remain taboo. Why? Why are we not shedding light on the fact that as many as 26 percent of all pregnancies and up to 10 percent of clinically recognized pregnancies end in miscarriage? In other words, why are we not telling other women that they're not alone on their journey?

Before you dive into this section on fueling your body to be the best mom on the run possible, know that whatever stage of motherhood you're currently in, when days feel desperately hard, you're not alone. Whether you're trying to conceive, or are joyfully yet fearfully pregnant, healing from delivery, in the midst of breastfeeding or mixing up some formula, or now navigating the half-day kindergarten schedule, know that you're far from alone. You are surrounded by a village of women, those who have gone before you and are here to light the path ahead.

NUTRITION TO FUEL 40 WEEKS

Pregnancy feels like an eternity, but technically, full-term gestation lasts between 37 and 42 weeks, with 40 weeks considered typical. The 40 weeks of pregnancy are divided into three trimesters, each lasting 12 to 13 weeks (3 months). Optimal nutritional status is critical before conception to prevent deficiencies and promote fetal well-being, and purposeful nutrition across all trimesters and throughout lactation has a significant impact on your future health, as well as on many facets of health for your child. The journey to motherhood requires a focus on foods before, during, and after 40 weeks to meet the demand for increased calorie and nutrient intakes to support the growth and development of the baby and to maintain your own health.

FUEL THE GROWTH: NECESSARY WEIGHT GAIN

It can be uncomfortable to anticipate weight gain during your pregnancy, but this addition is essential and purposeful. According to the American College of Obstetricians and Gynecologists, the recommended increase of approximately 30 pounds is distributed in the following manner: 7.5 pounds of actual baby weight, 1.5 pounds for the placenta, 2 pounds each of amniotic fluid, uterine growth, and breasts, and 4 pounds each for body fluids and blood. An additional 7 pounds for maternal stores of fat, protein, and miscellaneous nutrients are also included.

The amount of weight gained impacts the health of your baby and your own well-being during and after pregnancy. Ignoring the recommendation to gain adequate weight increases the risk for preterm birth, low-birth-weight infants, and difficulty initiating breastfeeding. Gaining too much weight also carries risks, such as delivering a baby weighing over 4,500 grams (around or over 10 pounds) and possibly requiring a cesarean section. Too much weight gain also can result in difficulty losing weight after pregnancy and a heightened risk of gestational diabetes and hypertension.

The right amount of weight gain during pregnancy varies for each woman and is based on your starting weight as well as your doctor's recommendations. General recommendations are outlined below. (Be sure to ask your doctor to help you determine the right amount of maternity weight gain for you.)

RECOMMENDATIONS FOR WEIGHT GAIN DURING PREGNANCY

Pre-pregnant BMI	Total weight gain (lbs)	First trimester gain (lbs)	Second and third trimester weekly gain (lbs)
UNDERWEIGHT: BMI <18.5	28–40	1.1 to 4.4 lb weight gain during the first trimester or as recommended by your physician to meet total weight gain recommendation	1 (1.0–1.3)
HEALTHY WEIGHT: BMI 18.5–24.9	25–35		1 (0.8–1.0)
OVERWEIGHT: BMI 25–29.9	15–25		0.6 (0.5–0.7)
OBESE: BMI >30	11–20		0.5 (0.4–0.6)

Every ounce you gain during pregnancy has a purpose, so build your new self wisely. You'll need to add nutrition above and beyond that which you consumed prior to becoming pregnant, to achieve your recommended weight gain goal as well as to replenish any energy expended in exercise and to preserve your own stores while accounting for your baby's needs. Grab nutrient-rich foods that agree with your system and don't cause nausea, vomiting, and/or food aversions. As the baby takes more and more space in your body, your ability to fit foods into your stomach will decrease, so be sure to make your calories work for you, prioritizing nutrient-rich foods and decreasing indulgent empty-calorie *sometimes* foods. Choose extra calories from colorful whole foods that are high in protein, vitamins, and minerals.

Wondering how much to add throughout gestation and lactation? Here's a general guide.

ESTIMATED CALORIE NEEDS DURING PREGNANCY AND LACTATION
FOR WOMEN WITH HEALTHY PRE-PREGNANCY WEIGHT

Stage of pregnancy	Estimated changes in daily calorie needs after fully accounting for exercise plus pre-pregnancy needs	What's that look like?
FIRST TRIMESTER	Fully account for exercise plus 0–100 calories	—Serving of Greek yogurt for protein, calcium, vitamin D. —Fortified cereal with milk and fresh fruit for folic acid, calcium, energy. —Apple with 1 teaspoon peanut butter for healthy fats and fiber. —Cheese stick and crudités for calcium, protein, and fiber.
SECOND TRIMESTER	Add 300–400 calories	—Half sandwich: whole grain bread with grilled chicken and fresh veggies for energy and filling fiber and protein. —Bowl of oatmeal with dried fruit, nuts for healthy fats, potassium, energy, and fiber.
THIRD TRIMESTER	Add 450–500 calories	—Pasta topped with grilled veggies and chicken for energy and vitamins and minerals. —Baked sweet potato topped with diced apple, butter and cinnamon for vitamin A, fiber, and energy. —Brown rice stir-fried with veggies and tofu for plant-based protein, fiber, and vitamins and minerals.
POSTPARTUM RECOVERY AND LACTATION	Add calories to support recovery and healing as well as milk production. Calorie recommendations account for desired energy deficit to facilitate weight loss.	Focus on protein, hydration, vitamin and mineral intake to create nutrient-rich milk while protecting your stores.
LACTATION DAY 1 THROUGH THE FIRST 6 MONTHS	Add 300–350 calories	Stay hydrated across the day, adding in milk/fortified nut milks, water, and juices, and rehydrate with electrolyte-rich beverages post-exercise. Add in lutein for brain and eye development with an omelet of eggs plus green leafy veggies plus corn.
LACTATION SECOND 6 MONTHS	Add 400–450 calories	As your workouts increase, add protein for recovery and satiation. Recover, refuel, rehydrate with: protein smoothie made with whole milk, whey protein, kale/spinach, frozen berries and bananas, peanut butter.

MEAL PLAN FOR TWO

I'm not one for being told what to eat and when, but when you're balancing a million other life choices as well as navigating countless medical appointments, having a loose guide on what to eat can be helpful.

Start with your current intake and build upon it to account for the energy burned during activity and additional calories to support your new needs plus baby's. Prioritize protein, natural color from fruits and vegetables, and plenty of fluids. Increase fluid intake to at least 8 to 10 cups per day, adding more to account for sweat losses. Your urine should be light yellow in color, but don't be alarmed if your prenatal vitamin impacts the color. If it's neon, simply recheck the color at other times of day.

For food and energy, consider the guidelines based on general population needs and build upon these recommendations as needed to account for sweat sessions and energy demands of your workout load:

First trimester and pre-pregnancy	Second trimester	Third trimester
MILK AND MILK PRODUCTS		
2 cups (teenagers) 4 cups (adults)	4 cups (teenagers) 6 cups (adults)	4 cups (teenagers) 6 cups (adults)
MEAT, OTHER PROTEIN		
2 servings, total 4 ounces	3 servings, total 6 ounces	2 servings, total 4 ounces
BREADS AND CEREALS		
6 servings (enriched, fortified, or whole grain)	6 servings (enriched, fortified, or whole grain)	6 servings (enriched, fortified, or whole grain)
FRUITS AND VEGETABLES		
5 servings, including a vitamin C source daily; a vitamin A source every other day	5 servings, including a vitamin C source daily; a vitamin A source every other day	5 servings, including a vitamin C source daily; a vitamin A source every other day

MOM ON THE RUN: TIPS AND TRICKS

Staying active during pregnancy is not impossible (or easy or predictable). Gait and weight are unlikely to change considerably during the first trimester, shielding you from the lower back pain or misalignment problems that are common complaints before delivery. Still, you may have to deal with other unforeseen symptoms such as fatigue, nausea and vomiting (morning sickness), food cravings or aversions, mood swings, constipation, frequent urination, or other unpleasant associations of pregnancy.

> **Pro Tip:** *Experts recommend pregnant and postpartum women engage in at least 150 minutes (for example, 30 minutes a day, 5 days a week) of moderate-intensity aerobic physical activity per week during and after pregnancy. It is best to spread this activity throughout the week. Many athletes find this baseline to be just the starting point of what is possible across 40 weeks.*

Pregnancy can affect your daily schedule, energy availability, and overall willingness to get out of bed in the first place, let alone lace up your running shoes. Some 70 to 85 percent of pregnant women experience morning sickness (morning, noon, and/or night), so afflicted pregnant runners need to be diligent about getting in enough fuel and fluids.

Meet your increased energy needs by opting for smaller, calorie-rich meals and plenty of nutrient-dense snacks throughout the day. This approach works wonders in early pregnancy if you're battling GI distress and during the third trimester, when you fill up quickly due to limited space. At any time, if you simply can't stomach solids, grab fruit and veggie smoothies or shakes with whey protein added in for additional calories and nutrients.

PRIORITIZE PROTEIN: Most women need at least 70 grams of protein each day, and pregnant athletes logging miles and crushing workouts need more. Include 15 to 30 grams at meals and snacks, keeping it simple by topping your salad or sandwich with just a few more slices of roasted chicken or steamed fish, hydrating with skim milk rather than water, or adding mild-flavored vanilla protein powder to smoothies, shakes, baked goods, waffles, and pancakes.

HERE ARE SOME NUTRIENTS TO WATCH: Pay close attention to intake of folic acid, a B vitamin that may help prevent neural tube defects, which are neurological disorders related to malformations of the spinal cord, such as spina bifida. These malformations result in severe birth defects that are unique to each individual and have no cure. Find folate in legumes and leafy greens and folic acid in fortified grains and supplements. Top off your intake with a doctor-recommended prenatal vitamin (typically containing at least 400 micrograms of folic acid), as it can be difficult to get the recommended amount from food alone.

Your need for calcium and vitamin D is also heightened during pregnancy. Your future superstar is being built from the ground up, requiring calcium for every single tiny bone in his or her body, and if you skimp, he or she won't! *You* will be left with a deficit, as the fetus pulls from your stores, setting you up for a deficiency and at risk for injury and osteoporosis. Consume at least 1,000 milligrams a day from a mix of calcium-rich foods including milk, yogurt, cheese, and calcium-fortified nut milks and orange juice, plus supplements as needed. Couple calcium intake with vitamin D, the sunshine hormone essential to baby's development. Amazingly, a mother's vitamin D status has been linked to her child's handgrip strength and even percent lean mass during his or her preschool years.

TAKE CARE OF YOUR TEETH: Unfortunately, many moms suffer from heartburn and may turn to calcium-rich antacids to fight it. These antacids may contain hidden sugars and increase the risk of cavities. Hormonal changes during pregnancy can also make your gums vulnerable to plaque, leading to inflammation and bleeding. So prioritize brushing your teeth and the use of oral rinses as recommended. After all, you'll be busy enough squeezing in a workout without also squeezing in extra visits to the dentist!

DON'T SKIMP ON IRON: Female athletes are often low in iron, and during pregnancy, iron needs increase significantly. During the first two trimesters of pregnancy, iron-deficiency anemia increases the risk for preterm labor, low-birth-weight babies, and infant mortality, and can even predict iron deficiency in infants after four months of age.

The prenatal vitamin you're taking for folic acid should also include iron (most all prenatal supplements meet 100 percent of your daily requirement of 27 milligrams per day).

To boost intake and enhance absorption, pair iron-fortified foods with a side of foods rich in vitamin C. (Vitamin C and iron have a relationship akin to that of calcium and vitamin D.) If you are suffering from iron-deficiency anemia, talk to your doc about supplementing even further, as some women have found they need 60 milligrams a day (or more) to resolve the anemia.

GET GOING WITH FIBER AND FLUIDS: Pregnancy-related slowdowns in the digestive system make you more likely to feel full and stay full hours after eating a meal. Additional iron can exacerbate this common concern. Fight constipation, help prevent late-stage hemorrhoids, and hasten gut motility with fiber, warm liquids, and extra fluids. Remember to give yourself extra time to use the facilities (multiple times, trust me) before heading out the door. That teeny-tiny person pressing against your bladder may force you to now plan your running route around rest stops, but being well hydrated is important for your health and baby's too.

HEIGHTEN HYDRATION: Adequate fluids can hold hunger and cravings at bay, assist in building new tissue, aid digestion, and form amniotic fluid. Aim for at least ten 8-ounce glasses a day (boost your intake by including soups, broths, Popsicles, and juices too), and if you perspire heavily, compensate for these fluid losses. Sip fluids early and often, and add in electrolytes as needed to maintain fluid balance. Into the third trimester, maintaining adequate fluids is paramount; contractions (without labor) can be triggered by dehydration.

> **Pro Tip:** As week 40 draws near (I get it, you thought it would never arrive), stock up the precious commodity of sleep. Dine light and early to promote better sleep, facilitate easier digestion, and avoid discomfort and heartburn. Instead, enjoy your biggest meal midafternoon; follow this up with a light dinner and small snacks when needed.

Oh, and while you're adding in the above foods and nutrients, steer clear of these baddies:

Caffeine-laced chews, gums, gels, energy drinks: Caffeine is a stimulant and diuretic linked to potential poor pregnancy outcomes. Experts recommend reduced intake of less than 300 milligrams a day, the equivalent of 2 to 3 cups of coffee.

Alcohol: Imbibing during pregnancy, especially in the first few months of pregnancy, may result in negative lifelong behavioral or neurological consequences in the offspring. No safe level of alcohol consumption during pregnancy has been established.

Certain fish: While fish are rich in protein and omega-3 fatty acids, some varieties are on the no-no list due to their mercury content. Avoid shark, swordfish, king mackerel, tilefish, and white (albacore) tuna (the latter of which should be limited to 6 ounces a week). Opt for shrimp, salmon, catfish, and pollock instead.

Deli meat: To avoid the risk of listeriosis (a food-borne illness that may cause flu-like symptoms and can lead to miscarriage, stillbirth, and premature delivery), you'll need to skip luncheon meat and hot dogs unless cooked, unpasteurized milk and foods made with unpasteurized milk, pâtés and meat-based spreads, refrigerated smoked seafood, raw and/or undercooked seafood, sushi, eggs, and meat.

Postpartum Nutrition

Welcome to the world of motherhood, full of joy and hilarity and mixed with a fair amount of guilt and confusion. Don't feel guilty if you're already dreaming of recapturing your identity as athlete but not quite certain how to attain your pre-pregnancy shape and weight. Deep breaths. Lots of patience will be needed postpartum. By incorporating healthy nutrition habits, exercising once you are medically cleared, and breastfeeding if you and baby are able, you will rapidly return to pre-baby shape. Remember, of all the amazing and intense anatomical and physiological changes you experienced through the previous months, the most significant of these were wholly related to weight gain that happened over nine months. And this same weight will be shed across sweat sessions, healthy eating, and a bit of time.

How long will it take you to get back to the sport you love and back to pre-baby weight? It depends on many factors, including genetics, age, pre-pregnancy weight, lifestyle, stress, and for many, even managing postpartum depression. The most consistent predictor of the total amount of time needed to shed baby weight is the total amount of weight gained over nine months.

Give yourself a break; it takes time and work, but the weight *will* come off and some of it quite quickly. Hours post-delivery, you'll shed approximately 10 pounds: losses of amniotic fluid and the placenta, plus the actual weight of your newborn baby. The image you see in the mirror will look different once you've delivered. Your core will have to readjust in the days after birth. Resist wanting to pummel those who ask you a week after delivery, "When's the baby due?" Been there, navigated that! A return to your former abs takes time. Some of the additional pounds will disappear in the first weeks as you shed additional fluid, including IV fluid infused during labor.

Pro Tip: *The average uterus is a superstar. It takes only six weeks to return to its original size despite being stretched to the max through the preceding nine months!*

If you choose to breastfeed, most experts agree that breastfeeding will burn/require 500 calories a day, with the added benefit of accelerating the tightening of your uterus and related core. Don't put extra stress on yourself about the timeline of your weight loss or your ability/choice to breastfeed, because not every woman is able or interested in breastfeeding and whatever you decide, the weight *will* come off regardless of how you feed your baby.

Let's Talk Lactation

Worried that weight loss and a return to sport will diminish your milk production and quality? When you pay careful attention to nutrition, hydration, and overall recovery, you can rest assured. Research shows that active women can maintain high-quality milk production supportive of infant growth while also maintaining slight caloric deficits even when accounting for the energy requirements of exercise. New moms coupling breastfeeding with activity will gain cardiovascular fitness and a faster return to their pre-pregnancy self. But managing to breastfeed while continuing with your sport is no easy task. Stephanie Bruce, who navigated two pregnancies in close succession plus a quick return to a high level of training, found that as her mileage increased, her milk supply tanked. And while it wasn't always feasible to breastfeed for the duration intended, she figured out ways to make both sport and lactation happen.

Find a regimen that works for *you*. Stephanie consumed fluids and a Picky Bar during feeding to keep her hydration and energy levels high as well as her milk production on point. She'd train and then, after a long session, feed her son, or if the prescribed workout was long, she'd pump. During the whole period, she gradually ramped up her mileage slowly, continuously listening to her body, backing off when needed.

> **Pro Tip:** To be on top of your (lactating and exercise) game, think through nutrition and fluids 24/7 in order to fire on all cylinders. Fuel up and recover with nutrient-rich and energy-dense foods. As baby and lactation pull from your stores, if you fail to replace nutrients, nutritional deficits can occur and increase your risk of injury, illness, and/or future health consequences.

Replace fluid losses post-workout to assure milk production. Hydrate before, during, and post-workout, sipping on water, protein shakes, and milk, adding in electrolytes to fight diuresis and support fluid retention.

DEAR YOUNGER, HUNGRY ME: STEPHANIE BRUCE

A formidable road racer with a marathon PR of 2:29, Bruce is also mom to sons Hudson and Riley, wife to speedy Ben Bruce, and the co-founder of Picky Bars. She's done it all from navigating body criticism to breastfeeding while running high mileage. Refreshingly wise and transparent, Bruce explains that life itself can be challenging and uncomfortable. But this discomfort makes you stronger and builds your courage so that when it's time to stand up for what you really believe in, you're strong enough to do so.

Dear Younger, Hungry Steph,

Good job. You have navigated the unknown complexities of your relationship with food very well. [You grew] up in a household with three brothers, all involved in sports, so food has been for fuel, for fun, and for gatherings. You got your period naturally around the age of thirteen/fourteen. Your body grew as it should. During high school you were on the softer side in the athletic arena, and it suited you well. You stayed healthy almost your whole high school career. You tried your hardest in running, didn't win all the time, actually rarely ever, but you learned how to work hard. You learned food was for fueling your body's needs and activities. There were times you perhaps had a little too much fast food, but you were being a kid. You were exploring and navigating your relationship with food.

At one point you attempted to give up dessert for your track season just so you could feel more dedicated. But it wasn't about calories, it was about replacing dessert for a healthier, more nutrient-dense option. You will carry this mantra into adulthood and into your future professional running career.

Here's where the path you began as a teenager led you to now:

I don't count calories but over the years have developed a healthy sense of listening to my body and knowing what it needs or is lacking. My weight doesn't fluctuate more than 3 to 4 pounds in a given training cycle. I get my period regularly every month naturally. I gave birth to two beautiful and healthy boys. They weighed 8 and 9 pounds, yikes! I do not get hurt very often. This information tells me I'm fueling pretty well and have done so for years.

—I do drink wine during training, maybe two to three times a week. I used to give it up as my race approached, but honestly I don't anymore.

—My go-to principle of nutrition is a protein smoothie after every workout and long run. Within 30 minutes of finishing.

—I eat pretty similarly on most days because it's the cumulative effect of training that we fuel for. I may aim for more protein on really hard workouts and lifting days, but my carbohydrate consumption is high all the time because of how many miles I'm running.

The sport that I am in can be a very dangerous and slippery slope. It is easy to compare yourself to others and even compare yourself to your previous self. But know this: Our bodies change. All the time. And it's natural and necessary. Our bodies are actually really intuitive and intelligent and know what's best.

So keep your heart open. Keep your stomach listening too. Block out any thoughts that tell you that you need less and you need to look a certain way or like someone else. There is only one you. You have only one body. Don't talk shit about it, and treat it well. Food is fuel. Fuel to train. Train to win!

Love Your Future Self,
Steph

EXERCISE RECOMMENDATIONS FOR MOM ON THE RUN

The number of miles I traversed—sometimes foolishly, often in an unsightly, slow, and painful manner—through three successful pregnancies: 1,276 miles, 890 miles, and 1,400 miles. This doesn't even touch the number of miles covered in attempts to run away from the darkness of *un*successful pregnancies. Exercise is one of the most powerful tools we can utilize to find peace and a connection with our true self, but during pregnancy, this tool is challenged. Temporary but substantial changes to every system in the body, from cardiovascular to musculoskeletal to endocrine and beyond, all impact your ability to enjoy the sweat sessions you crave.

But don't stop moving. Available research points to exercise as a tool to improve the health of both the mom and the baby. *Available research* is the key term here, because even in a society with more than 75 million women of childbearing age and a significant uptick in the number of girls and women participating in sport, little is known empirically about the risks and benefits of exercise during pregnancy. The research available on pregnant athletes is primarily from case studies and anecdotal in nature, given our collective desire to protect vulnerable research populations and the inherent risk and ethical considerations that surround research having to do with pregnant women and infants.

As a result, while running, cross-training, swimming, or sweating as a mom-to-be, you're bound to receive tons of unsolicited negative advice. The concern about whether women should exercise during pregnancy harkens back to the perceived fragile nature of women, enhanced by tons of unknowns. Consequently, all women, regardless of fitness level, are given similar advice: take it easy; keep your heart rate low; stay lightly active; accumulate approximately 150 minutes of activity across the week.

When asked if it's possible to do more, practitioners are limited to relying primarily upon expert opinion, anecdotal reports, and a handful of case studies rather than data from large clinical trials. In a recent journal article, Dr. Lauren Borowski and her colleagues note that perhaps the most significant consequence of this lack of data is the resultant protectionist nature of perinatal counseling, advising women to play it safe by not playing at all. Patients are advised "against performing a certain type or intensity of exercise not because it is known to have negative health consequences, but simply because any health consequences, if they exist, are unknown." The authors indicate that not only will playing it safe result in a potential decline in optimization of bone health, cardiovascular health, mental health, and protection against diabetes and metabolic syndrome, but also women miss substantial benefits such as avoiding excessive weight gain, gestational diabetes, gestational hypertension, preterm birth, cesarean sections, and even lower birth weight.

Progressive experts and athletes are pushing this discussion in a better direction. They remind us that putting a fit athlete on the sidelines for 40 weeks does much more harm than good. They've observed that when compared to the general (that is to say, mostly sedentary) population, female athletes who keep training—to a certain extent—as they did prior to conceiving maintain a healthy weight and their baby is born healthier.

But what if you can't exercise or simply don't want to? Certainly women under a doctor's orders not to exercise should *not* ignore their doctor's orders. Some conditions necessitate no to low levels of activity, limited stressors, even complete bed rest. You may not have envisioned a phase of life where you couldn't be active, but doctor's orders in this situation are critical. Keep in mind that this phase of life is short lived, and given time, you'll return to your fit self.

For others, who simply don't feel the need for speed, finding some activity that can keep you moving is a good idea. Should running become unenjoyable or uncomfortable, try swimming or walking. If you're a contact sport athlete, you'll need to find a lower-risk activity. Continuing to move *matters*. When we consider the health of female athletes who suddenly stop exercising and become detrained, the prognosis is worse than that for a sedentary pregnant women who doesn't exercise at all. You're effectively going backward, significantly altering your body's normal metabolic state, blood volume, even exercise-enhanced metabolic control. This forced inactivity places a new kind of stress on an already hardworking system.

If you worry about going too hard, it's unlikely to happen. "If you're a female athlete, you need to continue being a female athlete," says Stacy Sims. "Your body inherently will not let you go anaerobic. You'll become too uncomfortable and unable to hit anaerobic capacity because you can't breathe as heavy, you can't hit high intensities. Your body simply will not let you." So don't allow that Dri-FIT to gather dust for 40 weeks. Do what you can when you can and as much as you can. Your amazing body is built to support you.

Fitting It In

Being an athlete is far from easy. Add pregnancy or a kid or two to the equation, and finding the motivation and time for your beloved sweat sessions can feel damn near impossible. It's not the task at hand that gets harder, although the aging process doesn't exactly help. Being a mother runner is hard because the process of simply showing up gets harder. The road to reclaiming your athletic identity, your me time, your desperately needed mental release, and ultimately your best health is a bumpy one. Even the women who flawlessly navigate sport and motherhood find it to be an ever-evolving process. Winner of the first-ever women's Olympic marathon, Joan Benoit Samuelson, always describes her storied running career in two distinct phases: Before Children and After Diapers. Stephanie Bruce recounts that returning to running after childbirth involved an uphill battle as she worked to repair her core and pelvic floor, healing from diastasis recti, which can wreak havoc on stability and drive injury.

When I asked Bruce, who has more titles and job descriptions than seems humanly possible, how she balances being an athlete with being a mom and a wife, with being herself, she unabashedly explains: "I decided it was okay to have other passions. This means allowing yourself to hustle and enjoy the process. This means being brave enough to ask for help and not needing to ask for permission. This means divvying up the load. Taking away the stigma of putting everyone else first. Ask yourself, *Why can't* I *be first?*" Bruce is refreshingly right. So follow her lead, reignite your passion, and dust off your drive. You show up for everyone else, it's time to show up for you. You're a better mom when you take a moment for you. You're a better role model when you take time for your health. It's time to stop playing understudy or settling for second best. Go grab that leading role.

BUILD THE STRUCTURE, BUT NOT WITH FAD DIETS

An Intro to Fad Diets

Most fad diets have little to offer athletes. While I have seen some of these plans help certain athletes slim down, reduce their cholesterol, and cut out empty-calorie junk, for the vast majority of folks, diets leave a wake filled with hunger pangs and nutrient deficiencies.

But diet trends are everywhere. You can't scroll through social media or stroll a grocery store aisle without being bombarded by them. So it's important to understand what they're all about.

Yes, science-based and proven approaches to support weight loss or health improvements do exist. (I took a deeper dive into weight loss and health improvements in *Sweat. Eat. Repeat.*) I've employed these plans in health-seeking adults needing some guardrails, and I've used the keto diet to fuel ultramarathoners, help kids fighting epilepsy, and aid adults with appetite control or cognitive focus. But if you're a serious lifelong athlete, your best bet is to assemble a toolbox with various eating approaches that you can rely upon across different phases of your life. Most restrictive diets are about quick fixes and false promises. You just can't last fueled by foods you despise and longing for foods you love.

By now you're beginning to understand that this book is not written to promote false promises or easy fixes. Achieving your best self is more marathon, less sprint. That said,

> **Pro Tip:** At its core, the word *diet* refers to the kinds of food that a person habitually eats. For the purposes of this discussion, *diet* refers to prescriptive (or restrictive) approaches to eating and popular commercial schemes (for example, low carb or paleo) that proliferate in the media, on food packaging, and in conversation.

commercial diets do have some valuable elements that you can draw on as you work to build a lasting way of eating that helps you achieve your athletic goals.

What's Trending Now?

Some 43 percent of Americans ages eighteen to eighty reported trying a specific diet or eating pattern in the last year, with the practice increasing from 14 percent to 36 percent to 38 percent from 2017 to 2018 to 2019, respectively. Why diet? Given the staggering numbers of overweight and obese adults in the United States, the most common motivator for those who choose to adopt a new diet is the desire to lose weight and do so quickly. This desire for weight loss is trailed closely by a desire to feel better and have more energy (claimed by some 40 percent of those following diets). Still others seek improvements in physical appearance, and the desire to prevent future health issues rounds out the list of the top motivating factors.

As a dietitian, I totally understand these motivations. I am on board with anything that improves long-term health, and the desire to feel more energized is a worthy one. I'll argue that thoughtfully designed, purposeful nutrient-rich choices throughout your day can move you toward any or all of the above. In recent years, low-carb dieting, intermittent fasting, and clean eating have all gained steam. These plans tend to facilitate weight loss not because they do some metabolic magic trick, but simply because they limit calories.

After all, if your low-carb plan forbids bread, and you once lived off bagels and baguettes, there's a good chance your daily calorie intake will plummet and you'll lose weight. However, you'll also be scrambling to fill the void with proper nutrients.

Still, let's take a fresh look at some of these diets. After all, your nutritional needs and goals might line up with the principles of a popular diet, and your training partners, roommates, and colleagues may be talking about them. Sometimes these prescriptive plans help because whether you're a fitness enthusiast, an elite athlete, or an aspiring superstar, each one of us is bombarded with food options, commercials, and #foodporn 24/7. When we get overwhelmed, busy, or stressed, we sometimes want—even need—nutritional guardrails to help us stay on course. After all, decision fatigue is no joke.

Most conventional diets eliminate certain food groups or ingredients, or restrict eating to specific times of the day. These approaches often take away your control over what you put on your plate. For some of us, following these plans leads to feelings of accomplishment and empowerment. And because these approaches limit or eliminate junk calories, they might even support better control over health, appetite, and weight. But for some people, diets are the first step on the path toward restrictive intake, RED-S (see page 224), and dark days ahead. Before considering one of the following plans, know that they're not magic. Not all of them lead to performance or health improvements. And if you're prone to restriction or tend to pin your self-worth on your ability to follow a certain meal plan or daily calorie goal, these plans are *not* the best choice for you.

There is no "perfect diet" for everyone, forever. An eating strategy that works within the constraints of your current schedule, training, and goals may not work for you in a year. And that's okay. Our bodies, lifestyles, and goals will all evolve over time. The best diet for you at any given moment will be the one you can stick with and the one that helps you build a better relationship with food.

A DEEP DIVE INTO DIETS YOU'RE HEARING ABOUT

Intermittent Fasting

Designing your day around windows of time in which you are permitted to eat is nothing new. After all, people have fasted for religious reasons for eons, and you've likely had "nothing to eat or drink after midnight" in advance of an early morning lab draw or surgery. More recently, intermittent fasting, or IF—the concept of going without food for set periods of time and then eating only during a specific window—has become a popular weight-loss tool. Clinical research and anecdotal reports support claims of weight loss, mental clarity, an ability to focus on the task at hand without the distraction of eating, reductions in blood pressure, and improvement in blood glucose control and other markers of metabolic disease risk. But take note: the majority of fans in the IF camp are not athletes in heavy training, and you'd be hard-pressed to find a nutrition expert recommending IF for performance.

Here's what science says about this trend and some things to think about.

How (We Think) It Works

Intermittent fasting is more an eating schedule than a diet, and it purports to accelerate fat loss and muscle growth. The foundation is loosely based in both biology and human behavior. Circadian rhythms are involved in hormonal balance, including the appetite-regulating hormones leptin and ghrelin, and levels of each are influenced by the time of day. Studies suggest that consuming more calories earlier in the day aligns more closely with our circadian rhythms. But in real life we tend to consume the majority of our calories in the afternoon and evening. Our bodies rarely use copious amounts of calories before bedtime, instead storing them as fat. This excess calorie load in the evening can lead to elevated blood sugar, insulin spikes, and disrupted sleep.

Intermittent fasting purports to work around this problem, improve health, and prevent type 2 diabetes and obesity by narrowing the feeding window. On an intuitive level, this makes sense. If you tend to go overboard on calories after sundown (like most folks), this method might lead to weight loss.

Nutrient restriction from IF begins to deplete glycogen stores, and waning blood glucose levels tell the body that the energy from its favorite energy source, glucose, is close to gone. For survival, the body begins to transition to burning fat. The timing of this transition depends on how well fed you are heading into the fast, but generally this transition to fat burning happens anywhere from three to eight hours into fasting, and lasts for twelve to eighteen hours. During this time, the liver springs into action and breaks down glycogen to provide immediate energy and to maintain even blood sugar levels. Next, to keep up with the body's metabolic rate, whole-body fat breakdown increases. Thus there is an increase in levels of circulating free fatty acids, becoming a source of fuel for muscles.

Variations of Intermittent Fasting

Intermittent fasting can take a variety of forms, ranging from time-restricted fasting (restriction of calories during designated hours of the day) to alternate-day fasting (complete restriction of calories for entire 24-hour periods).

TIME-RESTRICTED FASTING/EATING: Restricts eating opportunities to a window of time—for example, 6:00 P.M. to 10:00 A.M. In this type of fasting, you spend the majority of the day in a fasted state. The example above would be called 16:8 fasting (16 hours fasting, 8 hours feeding). Time-restricted fasting can be as relaxed as 12:12 and as strict as 20:4.

ALTERNATE-DAY FASTING: This approach alternates strict zero-calorie fasting days (calorie-free liquids are allowed) with feast days, when you can eat and drink as much as you want.

MODIFIED FASTING: Sometimes referred to as 5:2 intermittent fasting, this variation calls for eating a regular diet five days a week and then limiting food intake to 20 to 25 percent of your calorie needs on two nonconsecutive days. So if you typically eat 2,000 calories a day, you'd eat 2,000 calories a day five days a week and about 500 calories or less on restricted days.

How Does Intermittent Fasting Impact Performance?

Is IF a good fit for athletes? Ask most sports dietitians, and you're likely to get a loud and resounding no.

The majority of research on IF revolves around Muslims fasting during Ramadan, a monthlong period when no food or liquid is consumed during daylight hours. Research has shown that athletes in high-intensity sports such as cycling, rowing, and running experience performance declines following a fast. When compared to fed athletes, fasted athletes experience losses in performance, such as peak power output and time to exhaustion for cyclists, time trial performance for rowers.

Still, some suggest that fasted exercise (whether going long and reaching empty or simply "training low" in the morning) might stimulate adaptations. I've personally experimented with this method and found that on light days and on days where the previous evening's meal was sufficient, it was easy to crank through a short, easy morning run with the added benefit of avoiding potential GI distress. But add in more miles and intensity and performance suffers. A firm believer in purposeful fueling, Olympian Ryan Hall adds, "I *never* ran empty. I am not a fan of depletion training at all. Marathon training is depleting enough. I am of the mindset that you fuel well for training and crush it so your body can grow and adapt from the higher level of training rather than from depleting it."

And so enters the other side of this argument: pre-exercise feeding boosts performance, strength, and speed better than fasting. This is a hard nut to crack given that most studies on IF and performance use short-term fasts and there is an adaptation phase (which is missing in most study designs but needs to be taken into account to allow for physiological adaptations). Therefore, the long-term effects (benefits? detriments?) of IF remain muddy.

With the goal of determining the effects of fasting versus pre-exercise feeding on continuous aerobic and anaerobic exercise, on performance during start-and-stop sports like basketball, soccer, or tennis, and on post-exercise metabolic adaptations, Aird and colleagues did a systematic review and meta-analysis of the effects of fasting (more than 8 hours) on performance. The findings suggest that short windows of fasting might not *hurt* performance. But there are no proven performance benefits of IF. So on game day, lean on the copious amounts of research proving the benefits of showing up to the starting line with that tank near full.

Is It Right for Female Athletes?

Nope. Dr. Stacy Sims, a global expert on female physiology and endurance training, notes that from a health standpoint, IF can be useful for the general population who are not very

> **Pro Tip:** For the nutrition and physiology nerds out there (did I see you raise your hand?), fasted exercise increases post-exercise circulating free fatty acids compared to fed exercise. These circulating fatty acids can be utilized as fuel during recovery while allowing glucose taken up by the skeletal muscles to be directed toward the resynthesis of glycogen (restocking energy stores).

active and commonly struggle with metabolic disease. However, for those layering IF on top of exercise, the benefits remain limited at best. In her book *Roar,* Sims explains that exercise in and of itself is a fasted state. Trying to perform taxing exercise in a heightened fasted state is a recipe for disaster.

Men and women have different responses to fasting, which is likely related to genetic adaptations to periods of scarcity. During short periods of fasting (12 to 24 hours), men experience an increase in metabolic rate, an increase in levels of growth hormone, a significant increase in utilization of testosterone, and even decreased risk factors for cardiovascular disease. Women don't respond to intermittent fasting in the same way. When survival and reproduction mode kicks in for the female athlete, metabolism slows and the body conserves energy and fat. That's not what we're going for.

> **Pro Tip:** In addition to disrupting hormones that impact many body functions, fasting can add more stress to an already underfed and overworked body, slow down the thyroid, increase the potential for fat storage, and disrupt the menstrual cycle.

Low-Carb Diets

Carbs are everywhere, and because carbs help humans run efficiently and effectively, that's a good thing for both survival and performance. But in the last thirty years or so, carbs have become a dirty word in our culture. More than a third of consumers across Europe and North America believe they should eat less bread, pasta, potatoes, and rice in the interest of weight and wellness. Even top-level athletes who need this efficient fuel for speed and distance often start nutrition counseling conversations by saying, "I need to cut carbs."

Most dietitians will tell you that carbs aren't intrinsically evil; it's *excess* carbs—overloading on *sometimes* choices like overly processed bagels and candy bars—that conspire to contribute to the epidemic of obesity.

Here's How Low-Carb Diets Work

Carbohydrates have increasingly gotten a bad rap and are blamed for rising obesity rates in the United States and globally. When asked which macronutrient contributes to weight gain, a recent weighted survey of American adults found that 48 percent of consumers point to sugars and carbs as being to blame. (Side note: Some 24 percent of consumers point to total calorie intake from all sources as equally likely to contribute to weight gain.) Such ostracization could be linked to the fact that as carbohydrate intake has increased over past decades, so have waistlines. But it's not that straightforward.

Over time, the average waistline has gotten bigger, and each diet has evolved to supply ever more calories from carbs. Alongside this increase, calorie intake rose while time spent exercising fell. This imbalance is the foundation for a significant uptick in prevalence of obesity. Data published by the Centers for Disease Control and Prevention from the National Health and Nutrition Examination Survey (NHANES) found that 42.4 percent of the U.S. adult population is now clinically obese. But when you look at the data trends, carb intake as a percentage of overall calories is actually on the decline while protein intake is increasing.

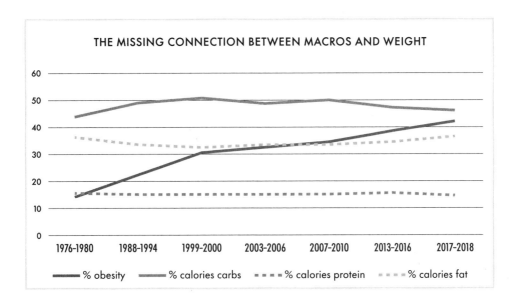

THE MISSING CONNECTION BETWEEN MACROS AND WEIGHT

▬▬ % obesity ▬▬ % calories carbs ▪ ▪ ▪ % calories protein ═ ═ ═ % calories fat

Let's back up a bit and define what "low carb" really means. Technically speaking, any low-carbohydrate diet is an eating plan supplying less than the acceptable macronutrient distribution range (AMDR) for carbohydrate. Established by the Food and Nutrition Board of the National Academy of Medicine, the AMDR provides guidance around intake of carbs, protein, and fat. These levels are based on decades of research (although I'm with the plethora of experts who suggest these levels need some tweaking based on more current evidence) and offer a range of macronutrient intake that supports reduction of chronic disease risk while allowing for adequate intake of essential nutrients. Most low-carb advocates limit intake to much less than the AMDR, encouraging 10 to 20 percent of calories from carbs, or approximately 20 to 100 grams per day. (In comparison, the Food and Nutrition Board established an acceptable distribution range for carbohydrate of 45 to 65 percent.)

The Science Behind Low-Carb Diets

The debate over the impact of low-carb diets on health and waistlines has been waged for decades, and it's not resolved yet. The evidence may be favorable for the general population of average, sedentary individuals. But for serious athletes, the effect of low-carb diets is clear: these plans don't support the growth and development of young athletes, high-intensity efforts, or overall performance.

For the general population, recent reports suggest that low-carb diets lead to poor outcomes and an increase in mortality. But I've seen many high-carb patients and clients suffering from severe inflammation and illness dramatically improve their health after reducing their carb intake and boosting their intake of high-quality proteins and fats. Studies suggesting poor outcomes tend to examine populations that were already at risk because of other lifestyle choices; individuals were more likely to smoke, exercise less, consume less fiber, and have a higher BMI.

If you're not in training but looking to manage appetite, reduce cardiovascular risk, triglycerides, and insulin levels, while also reducing the number on the scale, a low-carb diet can be a good solution. Likewise, if you want to see improvements in fasting blood sugar levels and your overall body composition. However, you can get many of these health benefits from other ways of eating.

Pro Tip: *Food groups go missing on low-carb plans. Watch out for nutrient deficiencies of vitamins A, B₆, C, and E, as well as thiamine, folate, calcium, magnesium, iron, potassium, and fiber. In addition, you might find yourself suffering from headaches and constipation; these are common complaints from people following low-carb diets.*

For athletes, the evidence is unequivocal: low-carb diets hurt performance and leave you open for injury. When it comes to performance benefits, your body loves carbs, craves carbs, for high performance. We are built to efficiently, effectively utilize carbs to fuel the brain and central nervous system and preserve muscle tissue (when carbs are adequate, protein needn't be a major source of fuel), and carbs even facilitate our ability to utilize fat as a fuel source.

Now you're probably wondering if you can turn to fat for fuel and find high performance on a very low-carb, fat-adapted diet (see the keto diet on the following page).

Over the years, I've seen many fat-adapted athletes perform at high levels without carbs, even at high intensity. These are more often male athletes on the ultra circuit who are looking for change because they suffer from GI distress or glucose intolerance, or they just can't take another sugary gel or syrupy sports drink. Conversely, I've worked with world-class Ironman athletes who are running full tilt and wondering if they can find yet another gear—and sometimes they can—by increasing their daily energy intake of calories from carbs, as high as 70 percent or more, during times of intense training.

There are few well-designed, female-forward studies that clearly link reduced carbohydrate intake to improved aerobic performance. For strength and physique sports, when increases in lean muscle mass due to increased protein intake are observed, or when shedding every ounce of excess fat and fluid is needed to make weight or to look good onstage, then keto and low-carb approaches can be a good fit (although not the only option). But in high-intensity endurance sports, and start-and-stop team sports, carbs are not only helpful but essential.

The Danger of Low-Carb Diets for Female Athletes

What happens when we layer exercise stress on top of the stress of denying our bodies carbohydrates? Stress hormones like cortisol rise even higher. As the demands of workouts (and those of life, if we're being honest) compound that stress and the sympathetic drive remains high, potentially reducing our ability to relax and depressing our thyroid activity, this can mess with your menstrual cycle.

This spike in cortisol from carb restriction can impact bone health and break down muscles, hurting performance and overall health, Stacy Sims says. It also impacts an already taxed immune system. "In the end, a low-carb diet compromises your ability to maintain high-intensity or prolonged periods of exercise and puts your body under exorbitant stress."

While carbs get the green light, quality and quantity still matter. As we age and our estrogen levels decline, our bodies become more sensitive to carb intake. Therefore, to boost performance and achieve an ideal body composition, many experts recommend consuming a diet rich in quality proteins and fats, with 40 to 45 percent of total calories from complex carbohydrates. I'll second this advice: For years I've aimed for 40 percent of daily calories from carbs, 30 percent from fats, and 30 percent from protein, with great success. I modify this plan as needed: if I'm into heavy training or a big race, I'll eat more carbs, while still keeping my overall health and body composition goals within sight.

In summary, carb restriction might be an option for the general sedentary population looking for weight loss, but for athletes looking for high performance, carb is the fuel you need to gain speed and go the distance.

Ketogenic Diet (Keto)

The ketogenic diet is actually not new; this high-fat, adequate protein, *very* low-carb approach has been used for decades to treat epilepsy and, more recently, metabolic syndrome and type 2 diabetes.

Here's the premise behind this diet. If carbohydrates are severely restricted, the body is forced to either find an alternate source of fuel or perish. Survival mode kicks in, and instead of being a carb-burning machine, relying on blood sugar for fuel and the pancreas and insulin to utilize said fuel, the body transitions to burning endogenous fat stores and exogenous dietary fat, while the liver creates a source of fuel known as ketones. When this happens, the body enters a metabolic state known as ketosis, in which its energy supply comes primarily from burning fat for fuel, translated into ketones. These ketones are used by the brain and muscle tissue as a fuel source to replace some of the needs originally supplied by glucose. (There is still a low level of circulating glucose available for essential functions that demand glucose as fuel.)

But given that for the past several decades, nutrition guidance has focused on strategies to match the body's finite carbohydrate stores to cover the distance or speed or demand of training regimens and competitions, it seems counterintuitive to pivot so far from proven performance fueled by carbs.

We've spent decades fine-tuning carb-loading protocols to optimize muscle glycogen stores. We've trained our gut to tolerate sickly sweet gels, chews, and sports drinks so we have a sustained source of carb during long runs and marathons. So why the fascination with fat-based fueling when we know carbs can enhance endurance performance, support motor recruitment, maintain pace, and keep our perception of effort and intensity as low as possible?

Keto diets appeal to athletes for a variety of reasons. For some, the diet holds the potential to fight inflammation, contribute to muscle health, and prevent exercise-induced fatigue. Others are lured by the potential to utilize all available sources of energy, especially fat, given that the body has a limited capacity to store carbs. Since even the leanest of athletes has stores surpassing approximately 16,000 grams of fat, many athletes are fascinated with the idea of tapping into the endless source to power performance.

The majority of keto studies don't allow time for adaptation and are based on small samples, but they do offer interesting insights. For example, a ten-week pilot study (n = 5; 4 women) exploring the effects of a keto diet on body composition, performance outcomes, and overall endurance found improvements in body composition and well-being, but not performance. Athletes reported a lull in energy, followed by a return to high levels of energy across workouts, but they struggled to easily undertake bouts of high intensity. All athletes increased their ability to use fat as a fuel source, even at higher exercise intensities. But as far as significant impact on performance, they got tired faster, and other performance metrics (VO_2 max, peak power, and ventilatory threshold) were impacted.

Before writing off keto, consider that, similar to the above study findings, ketogenic diets generally do result in improved well-being and body composition. Decreased performance, while significant at first, is also temporary and attributable to an inadequate adaptation period. Studies suggest full keto adaptation takes up to twelve weeks, and during this time, performance will flux as the body transitions to primarily burning fat for fuel. But if the body is given enough time to fully adapt, its ability to utilize fat for fuel and preserve muscle glycogen stores may be just intriguing enough to start building a ketogenic plate.

On your plate, keto looks like this: coffee blended with MCT oil and whipping cream, and a cheesy omelet topped with avocado and bacon for breakfast; a lettuce-wrapped burger for lunch; and a rib-eye steak topped with buttery sautéed mushrooms and spinach for dinner.

Ketogenic diets facilitate weight loss due to metabolic shifts and an overall reduction in calorie intake. Given the strict carb restriction, ketogenic diets do not allow for intake of empty-calorie high-sugar treats, nor do they allow for an overwhelming choice of foods. In addition, the removal of carbs leads to eliminating common blood sugar fluctuations that can increase appetite and hunger—side effects commonly reported on high-carb diets.

What Does the Science Say?

Definitions of a ketogenic diet can vary, but follow these general guidelines:

1. **VERY low carb:** Less than 20 to 50 grams of carbohydrate per day, or less than 5 to 10 percent of total daily calorie intake.

2. **Adequate protein to support lean body needs:** 0.45 to 0.7 grams per pound, or about 20 percent of daily calories.

3. **High fat:** Fats and oils supply the vast majority (70 to 75 percent) of daily calories.

4. **Keep it simple:** Consume at least twice the amount of fat compared to protein plus carb. For example, if you consume 100 grams of fat, eat less than 50 total grams of carb plus protein.

When it comes to weight loss and improvements in body composition, multiple studies have found keto to be effective short term and to produce weight loss across three to six months. While some studies suggest that following a keto diet for up to thirty-six months can provide better results than a low-fat diet, other studies have found that after the first few months of weight loss, dieters plateau.

When it comes to overall health, ketogenic diets can support improvements in cholesterol and inflammatory markers and reduction in chronic disease risk, sometimes as a result of significant weight loss.

Not all the research on the ketogenic diet is positive, and not all clinicians advocate for this restrictive approach to eating. While some individuals like keto because it allows them to eat some commonly forbidden foods, clinicians criticize the diet for severely restricting food groups and question its use as a long-term approach to health and wellness. Across my practice, I have seen this diet aid in weight loss and assist those struggling with chronic diseases, and even help athletes seeking fuel for the long run. But that's when these individuals were following a properly designed plan packed with variety and nutrients. I've also counseled plenty of clients through the side effects of keto diets (all of which can be prevented with careful planning), such as dehydration, electrolyte losses, fatigue, micronutrient deficiencies, and difficulty with making it work.

Keto for Athletes?

Remember, much of the data on keto comes from the overweight and obese population seeking accelerated and significant weight loss as well as improvements in blood glucose control and outcomes relating to type 2 diabetes. These types of studies don't typically translate to athletes who want to improve performance. Olympian Ryan Hall experimented with keto, and it went badly, quickly. "I played with keto for a bit and performed terribly . . . I could run a 6-minute pace all day burning fat, but when I needed to get down to race pace (4:45 per mile), I felt like I was stepping on the gas pedal and getting no acceleration."

The availability and capacity to use all fuels to support the demands of exercise (otherwise known as metabolic flexibility) is the holy grail for high-performance endurance athletes, explaining their continued fascination with strategies to better utilize the body's relatively unlimited fat stores. There is robust evidence that adaptation to a ketogenic low-carb, high-fat (LCHF) plan creates substantial cellular changes to increase the mobilization, transport, uptake, and oxidation of fat during exercise, even in elite athletes who specifically train to optimize fat oxidative pathways.

While the benefits of keto for serious athletes have yet to be fully examined, current research is mixed, suggesting it's likely not the right approach for athletes in high-intensity sports. So if you're looking to PR at your next track meet or totally own your next HIIT session, weigh the pros and cons of keto before jumping in.

Many athletes who have transitioned to a ketogenic diet during the off-season report improvements in body composition as well as other performance markers. Others find no performance improvements, quickly tire of limited food options, and ultimately crash and burn on fat-based fuel.

If you do decide to try out keto, know that it takes several weeks for your body to adapt. So don't wake up on Monday with a plan to start keto when you've got an important race on Friday.

Does Keto Work for Women?

Keto benefits and outcomes are different for men and women. In women, an increase in sympathetic or fight-or-flight response can take place, potentially causing upticks in anxiety, sleeplessness, and difficulty focusing. Such results can hamper an individual's recovery from workouts and negatively impact hormonal health, performance, and well-being. Conversely, many women report following a ketogenic diet with great success, reaping health, wellness, and performance benefits.

Large longitudinal keto studies on women are lacking, and there have been limited studies examining possible keto-related differences in energy metabolism between genders. Try to find athlete-centric, gender-specific data, and the evidence gets even more sparse. However, it has been established that there are gender differences in whole-body reliance on fat as fuel during exercise. In general, women use greater amounts of fat at submaximal intensities and have an ability to burn fat to a greater extent, even at higher exercise intensities, than men.

Virtually nothing has been more contentious in the nutrition world than specific approaches to eating, especially when it comes to carbohydrates versus fats. While low-carb diets, keto diets, and other variations on these themes may be dissimilar, it's entirely possible for them to arrive at similar end points. And while everyone is wondering which is better for performance, weight loss, or health, it needn't be an issue of either/or.

Rather than debate the efficacy of the various approaches, consider the similarities between them that support everybody. We can all agree that spending the whole day grazing on highly processed, sugary junk benefits no one. We can agree that vegetables are important to health and we should all consume more of these. Whatever plan you choose, it's a good thing to consistently eat less sausage and bacon and instead grab fatty fish, nuts, and avocados. Remember to consider the long-term viability and sustainability of any plan, choosing an option that works for you. And consider the why behind your plan; you're much more likely to stick with and enjoy a plate that helps improve what matters most to you.

DEAR YOUNGER, HUNGRY ME: RYAN HALL

There's reinventing yourself, transforming yourself, and then there's Ryan Hall. The U.S. record holder in the half-marathon (59:43), he became the first U.S. runner to break the one-hour barrier. He is the only American to run a sub-2:05 marathon (2:04:58 at the 2011 Boston Marathon). Ryan has represented the United States in the marathon after winning the 2008 United States Olympic Trials and placing tenth in the Olympic marathon in Beijing. He wasn't content to sit by and watch once he retired from the sport of distance running. Instead he turned into a strength athlete who's always pushing himself to see what the human body is capable of. He's also coach to his wife, Sarah Hall, and a mentor and advocate for his four daughters. He sounds in as a coach, runner, and father, and I'm honored to share his wise and moving advice.

Dear Younger Hungry Ryan,

"Find the middle path."

I know you hate the middle path. I know you love the extremes because the extremes are where you see the most instant and dramatic results. But here is the secret: every time you go after instant results, you trade long-term, optimal results. If you really want to see how good you can be in this sport, you must find the middle path.

The founder of Buddhism thought he could find enlightenment through extreme self-deprivation. Yet, after long periods of self-denial and self-inflicted starvation, he found this was not the way. He also lived in a palace with his every need met and his every physical craving satisfied, but this too did not yield enlightenment. He found enlightenment when he discovered the middle path between extremes of self-control and deprivation and extreme indulgence of the fleshly desires. Nutrition is the same way. It's really easy to think that getting optimal results happens only through dieting, perfect nutrition, or, as some believe, just eating whatever you want whenever you want. These extremes do not hold optimal results. Results lie in the middle.

The body operates in the here and now, so there are times when eating way more carbs than your body needs at the moment is necessary because you have a marathon the next day. Your body doesn't know what is coming, so there will be times you have to force it to take in the nutrition it is not craving. Similarly, there will be times post-workout and race when the body doesn't feel like taking in food. Again, you must give it the building blocks it needs to recover through nutrition so that it can restore itself.

Nutrition does matter. Nutrition will make a huge impact in how you perform. Similarly, if your goal is to optimize your performance, weight does matter. Carrying around even just a few extra pounds will negatively impact your performance. I wish that this was not the case. Now, I want you to hear me very clearly. This does not mean that you need to look like a Kenyan or an Ethiopian. I know you look at them and you look at you and it always makes you feel like you need to lose weight so you can look and perform like them. The truth is, if you look like them you will perform terribly, because you are not built like them. You have a bigger frame and need to carry around extra weight to support that frame. You need to find the weight you are strong and light at and make sure you are at that weight when your goal race rolls around. You need to be the weight you are performing the best at, and lighter is not always faster.

It is good to have your weight change throughout the year. You will not perform well if you are staying race-lean year-round. You need to put on weight in the off-season so that your hormones get back into a healthy state and your body can completely recharge all of its systems.

You will need to go through periods when you lean out. Do this in a healthy way. No more than 0.5 pounds per week, and DO NOT starve yourself to do this. Eat lots of healthy foods. Surround your workouts with carbs. Eat high-volume, high-fiber foods that nourish your body. Realize that this is not a sustainable diet. Once you reach race weight (ideally three weeks prior to your goal race), you need to up your calories in order not to continue to lose weight.

Equally important is finding a healthy way to put on weight after your goal race. Think about this period as a time to give your body beyond what it needs so that it can get back to a healthy state. I know you like to do this by doing endless doughnut-eating competitions and binge eating on as much sugar and fried food as possible, but this is not a healthy way to put on weight. It is absolutely okay to enjoy foods you don't often eat, but in moderation. When you find yourself going back for another doughnut, think of substituting a nice piece of fatty salmon that will hit that same craving for fatty foods but in a way that will be beneficial for your body.

Have lots of grace for yourself. Your nutrition doesn't need to be perfect, so when you fail, the goal is to "get back on the horse" as quickly as possible without beating yourself up about it. When you feel guilty for binge eating, take a moment to think to yourself, What would I tell my best friend if they were going through this exact experience? Have compassion for yourself in your weakness.

Find the middle path. Stay away from fad diets and extremes of any nature when it comes to nutrition, and know at what weight you are strong, light, healthy, and perform the best. Don't stay there year-round. See the extra weight you gain in the off-season as your "training weight" that will provide extra resistance to make you extra strong for your next race.

Most of all, enjoy your food and see it as it is: something to give us pleasure and to nourish our body so it can perform optimally. Eat as close to how

God made things as possible, and you will be in good hands. Have much respect and love for those who choose to eat differently from you and be inspired by their dedication to their beliefs. Lastly, remember that you need lots of energy to fuel you toward your goals. Food is measured in calories, and a calorie is a unit of energy. That energy is what you need to accomplish your goals. Calories are your friend, not something to slow you down. Eat up!

—Your Future Self

THE RIGHT FUEL AT THE RIGHT TIME

Ask a group of nutrition experts to sound in on the one thing they wish athletes did differently, and the vote will be nearly unanimous. "I wish they understood and valued the power of nutrient timing." Dana Angelo White, a sports dietitian and associate clinical professor of athletic training and sports medicine at Quinnipiac University, elaborated on this theme with a universal truth: "*When* you eat is as important as *what* you eat . . . especially across traveling and competition days. Proper timing can make the difference between optimal performance and a disappointing finish."

For health and longevity, *what* you eat absolutely matters. For performance, the w*hat* is joined by the *when*. You already know the how, the why, and the best sources of each macro. Nutrient timing simply quantifies the what and specifies the when. The amount and types of fuel needed to top off your tank, maintain your pace, and fully recover are dependent on the length, type, and intensity of the workout.

Why does it matter? The right fuel prevents fatigue and supports critical outputs of performance such as power, agility, strength, focus, and skill. The right fuel prevents dehydration, electrolyte and fluid imbalances, glycogen depletion, hyper- and hypoglycemia, GI discomfort, and other nutrition-related factors influencing performance and ultimately health.

Implementing the right timing of the right fuel can be the difference between hitting the wall early and not hitting it at all; between fully recovering from a tough workout and experiencing intense fatigue and delayed-onset muscle soreness (DOMS). In essence, the art of nutrient timing fuels your body so it can tackle whatever task you throw at it. With purposeful selection, food logging, and a little trial and error, you'll be on your way to determine what works best for you.

FUEL YOUR PERFORMANCE: BEFORE, DURING, AND AFTER FUELING STRATEGIES

S tarting and finishing a workout, race, or game with your faculties intact and a smile on your face takes some serious planning and lots of trial and error. Your ultimate goal is to find food, fluids, supplements (bars, chews, gels, powders) that agree with your gut and to ingest them in quantities that ensure you'll show up ready to compete, with the energy to cover distance and the power needed to chase down opponents and accelerate for as long as needed without hitting empty.

The amount of nutrition you'll need is complex and dependent on the event, the environment, how well you recovered from previous workouts, and even what phase of your menstrual cycle you're in. Consuming the right types and amounts of pre-workout fuel can reduce your rate of perceived exertion (RPE), effectively making your workout feel easier. By consistently consuming adequate carbohydrate before and often throughout your event, you stock up and maintain your energy stores, ultimately preventing premature fatigue from setting in before you reach the finish line or that final whistle blows. Here's how to master pre-workout and mid-workout fueling.

PRE-WORKOUT FUEL

When you think of lasting and healthy pre-workout energy, think carbs. These gems are a powerhouse of easily absorbed energy, driving muscles and ultimately powering the body through an activity-packed day. In her buildup to the New York City Marathon, Canadian distance runner and sports dietitian Rachel Hannah focused on eating more carbohydrates at optimal times. As a result, her energy levels and performance improved, along with her menstrual cycle health.

Kara Goucher adds: "By eating simple and pure carbs the night before a hard workout, you set yourself up for a great session the next day." So don't fear carbs; don't overlook this foundation of fueling. Without proper pre-workout priming, you may not be able to crank through even the lightest of workouts.

Rather than bonk miserably, research suggests you fuel up in the one to four hours pre-workout, paying attention to what works and what doesn't.

> **Pro Tip:** Write down what you chose, how much you ate, and whether it worked or didn't.

If you know you'll be going long without the opportunity to refuel, keep blood glucose and energy levels steadier by opting for slower-to-digest carbs rather than simple, sugary carbs.

DEAR YOUNGER, HUNGRY ME: RACHEL HANNAH

Talk about putting science into practice and using your own experiences to drive the potential of others. Rachel Hannah is as talented in translating nutrition science into performance as she is at pushing her limits as a Canadian distance runner. She's competed multiple times in the IAAF World Cross Country Championships, won the Canadian Cross Country Championships, and received a bronze medal in the Pan American Games marathon. During her time in sport, Rachel has personally dealt with underfueling, injuries, and setbacks, and as a registered dietitian, she works tirelessly to educate other athletes to avoid relative energy deficiency and instead fuel health and performance. She has vocally promoted the importance of nutrition and sounds in on how to identify low fueling and how to help your teammates and yourself find a way out of the darkness of injury and eating disorders.

Dear Younger, Hungry Rachel,

I wish I could have spoken kinder words to you. I know you heard a lot of negative inner dialogue over the years and at the peak of your competitive years as an elite distance runner. I wish this could have been balanced out with a voice that recognized how strong, resilient, and amazing you did during difficult times. Competing with the world's best women took its toll on you, and you certainly learned a lot about yourself in the process. With adversity come new learnings, and what a privilege it is to reflect and share this with the younger generation of athletes.

First, I wish you did not compare your body shape and size to those of other elite distance runners. You were self-critical, and this did not serve as an advantage. This was the root cause of the restrictive type of behavior you had for many years with food. You wanted to become smaller and look more like your competitors because you had body dissatisfaction. While your body got smaller and you performed well, your health took the back burner and suffered. You had incredible performances while not fueling your body properly, and the chase of the high feeling associated with accomplishment and feeling "fit" overtook the lows of disappointing races and health consequences from developing relative energy deficiency in sport (RED-S).

What I wish you knew back then was that it is okay to gain weight in between competitive seasons. In fact, it is very healthy to train at a higher body weight and then compete at a lower weight. This periodization of weight in the year would have helped your energy availability and bone health. Just how we must periodize our training, the same applies to nutrition. I wish you would have eaten more carbohydrates on workout and long-run days to fuel your body properly and had a specific plan in place instead of relying on hunger cues alone. You developed this mismatch in energy intake unintentionally some days and other days did it intentionally to remain at a lower body weight.

You should have researched more on just how dangerous it is to lose your menstrual cycle for extended time periods. This led to five stress fractures and a lot of time off from running, including missing your biggest competition, the Marathon World Championships. I would have told you to get to a place where you feel strong and fast but are also getting your menstrual cycle regularly, as this is essential for bone health.

Learning how to listen to your body and not always sticking to the training plan are actually very important for long-term development and success. This means when energy levels are low, taking a rest day or doing a shorter recovery run. You were too focused on "burning calories" and always sticking to what your coach said. The fatigue from training is created from a combination of factors, but clearly one reason for some workouts and long runs feeling harder than they should was low carbohydrate intake. I wish you had eaten more carbs on higher training volume/intensity days.

Upon reflection, you certainly learned a lot during the times off from *injury, including how to help improve bone density through regular men-strual cycles, and consume adequate calories, calcium, vitamin D, and the other bone-building nutrients. You learned how to change your body weight based on the season and eat more calories (specifically carbs) on higher training days. You are still able to do what you love for now, which is run. Nothing quite compares to the freedom of going out for a run. Improving at running requires consistency, which is much easier to do when one is taking care of the details to stay healthy and happy.*

—Rachel Hannah

HOW THE PROS STAY FUELED

Need some inspiration for what to eat before a workout or race? Here's what the pros eat before go-time:

KARA GOUCHER: The night before a race or a hard workout, Goucher aims for a mix of carbs and lean protein—for example, rice and sweet potatoes with a salad or a dish of sautéed veggies with chicken or fish. Knowing that the pre-race dinner might not offer familiar favorites, she says, "I look for simple carbs (rice/pasta/bread) and lean meat (fish/chicken)." Just in case, she never travels without instant oatmeal. "It makes me feel like I have something if I need it, and the oatmeal always digests easily in my stomach."

RYAN HALL: Find an easy-to-digest go-to meal or beverage with complex carbs, a simple source of protein, and a little healthy fat to stabilize the blood sugar, such as Hall's go-to shakes made with protein powder mixed with maltodextrin (30 grams of protein and 400 calories of maltodextrin) plus 1 tablespoon of coconut oil.

RACHEL HANNAH: Her go-to pre-run meal is oatmeal with banana plus half a Clif Bar on race day, plus coffee with milk. If there are 2½ or more hours before the workout, Hannah eats overnight oats made with milk or Greek yogurt plus fruit; this dish is a typical lunch on a workday with a hard afternoon or evening session planned after work.

DEENA KASTOR: With the goal of always exploring new foods and avoiding falling into an eating rut, Kastor doesn't have a specific go-to. Instead she aims for a colorful combination of carbs and protein like toast with butter and nutritional yeast, and a juicy peach. Or sometimes cashew pancakes with blueberries and syrup.

GRAYSON MURPHY: The night before a long and hard effort, Murphy opts for a filling dinner: a good mix of carbs, proteins, fats, and colors (she notes that actually this "pretty much sums up all of my dinners"). The morning of the race, she dines on a combination of oatmeal, banana, fruit, peanut butter, or toast.

MOLLY SEIDEL: Finding fuel that works has taken a bit of experimenting. The evening before a long effort, Seidel opts for rice and fish or potatoes and fish. Formerly fond of eggs, she now skips them due to an intolerance and instead sources protein and fat from toast and peanut butter or oatmeal and butter: "I've learned fat is really an important fuel, but I don't add too much right before a run or GI distress follows." Given that caffeine improves performance, Seidel always adds a cup of coffee.

DES LINDEN: Dinner the night before a long run often includes rice or pasta mixed with a bit of chicken or beef. She gravitates toward real, simple fare, choosing whole foods and home cooking over processed or fancy. She's a no-fuss flexible eater, and her pre-run choice is commonly an egg sandwich or toast topped with avocado or peanut butter and a full mug of coffee. (Linden's husband, Ryan, is the roaster behind Linden × Two, a company that makes specialty—and might I add delicious?—coffee.)

TATYANA MCFADDEN: Following a simple no-fuss relatively high-carb diet carries McFadden across intense training weeks of 150 to 200 miles. She might pre-fuel with a glass of nitrate-rich beet juice and espresso or eat whole grains some two hours before go-time. "Before a workout (or a race)," she says, "I do not eat much—usually a very bland carb along with hydrating with water and coffee. Wheelchair racers lean on their stomachs to get into a more aerodynamic position, so I cannot fill up completely."

TIME TO GET TECHNICAL: ADVANCEMENTS IN PRE-WORKOUT FUELING

For as long as I can remember, sports nutrition experts (myself included) fearful of hitting the ominous wall have been advising athletes to eat across the pre-workout hours, prioritizing adequate fuel at all costs. Those athletes who chronically interpret nutrition timing as "grab a bite immediately prior to a workout" face a train wreck. Yes, you can sometimes get lucky and find a banana on your way to the gym, but as the digestive system is not equipped to break down or absorb nutrients instantaneously, procrastinators risk running into serious trouble. Even if you can avoid severe GI issues, last-minute meals are bound to create GI distress like heartburn, diarrhea, and cramping without even supplying the energy needed to perform.

Forward-thinking experts are now uncovering additional reasons, besides mid-run discomfort and lost time at pit stops, that it may not be optimal to eat within an hour or two of the starting gun. Researchers using data from continuous glucose monitors (CGM), wearable technology initially developed to allow for real-time blood glucose monitoring in individuals with diabetes, have found that athletes who consume quickly digested carbs immediately prior to a workout commonly experience significant spikes and plummets in energy levels during the workout. Prior to having access to a CGM like the Abbott Libre

Sense Glucose Sport Biosensor, used with the Supersapiens app, clinicians and scientists could monitor athlete blood glucose levels but only at a few points in time and rarely mid-workout. We now know the impact of certain pre-workout fueling strategies and realize that loading up on carbs in the hour before a workout could be detrimental.

Here's how we think it works. After you consume carbs, insulin is secreted by your pancreas, responding to allow glucose to enter the cells, where it can be put to work. While primarily responsible for shuttling glucose from the bloodstream (that is to say, blood sugar) to cells and on to working tissues, insulin is also a fat-depositing hormone and can present difficulties with access to fuel stores during activity. When there is excess circulating glucose, insulin kicks into overdrive, eventually resulting in a rather severe valley known as rebound hypoglycemia, especially if insulin is shuttling glucose while your muscles are also requesting their own supply. Plummeting blood glucose values correspond with plunging energy levels. (This is akin to the "food coma" you may fall into after a large meal.) Luckily, if fuel choice and timing are tweaked, your performance needn't falter.

Blood glucose will peak at approximately 60 to 90 minutes (depending on the contents of the meal and your personal response to it), so if you eat immediately before a workout, your system is working to digest and perform, but this timing means that insulin is in the midst of responding to high blood glucose values, shuttling sugar (and likely storing fat, making it also inaccessible) at a time when you're desperately in need of some fuel.

Todd Furneaux, president and co-founder of Supersapiens, says the best fueling strategy is through proactive planning. Based on thousands of glucose data points, the greatest way to assure adequate and steady glucose is likely twofold:

1. The evening before a long workout, add a second dinner, a mixed small meal with slow-to-digest carbs, to prime your tank.

2. The morning of the race or workout, load up on carbs three to four hours out, giving yourself time to fully digest and stock glycogen. If you don't have this kind of time in the morning, there is a work-around. Hydrate as normal, but don't have food. Instead, during your active warm-up, add in a source of carbohydrate (such as a gel, an energy bar, or a sleeve of chews) to activate your GLUT4 glucose

transporter (which is a fancy way of saying this fuel will be transported). Thus glucose will be made available to power your performance without a spike, valley, and bonk.

Putting Science into Practice

When you load up with carbs just hours before a long run, you may be mentally ready to hit the road, but with insulin causing interference in the background, you will fail to find the next gear. There's fuel in the tank, but it's not as readily available as expected. I've found two successful strategies to prevent this. Both involve allowing adequate time to eat something.

Strategy 1: Mixed Meals

Fat, protein, and carbs are all absorbed by the body at different rates, and adding fat and protein to your pre-workout meal can help keep your energy levels stable. Add pre-workout protein—approximately 10 to 20 grams, depending on your size and your overall daily needs—and make this a permanent habit on your most grueling workout days and especially during the catabolic high hormone luteal phase of your cycle (see page 216). In addition to blunting blood glucose spikes and keeping energy levels steady, this protein boost will improve muscle protein synthesis and even help you recover faster. Use this mixed meal approach when you're pressed for time, when your workout is shorter than 90 minutes, and before start-and-stop team sports.

Strategy 2: More Time for More Carbs

When you have a longer or more intense workout—say, an event that's 90 minutes or more—or a shorter workout approaching race pace, you need plentiful fuel on board. Top off the tank with about 10 grams of protein and about 1.5 to 2 grams per pound (3–4 g/kg) of carbs about 4 hours before go-time. This will stop any pre-event hunger and allow your system to fully digest and absorb the fuel, storing some as muscle and liver glycogen for later and circulating the rest, providing a performance-ready blood glucose level, primed to elevate your energy levels and pace, rendering you ready for a peak performance.

TIME TO GET TECHNICAL: CRANKING WHILE CUTTING CALORIES

When it comes to performance and health, calorie cutting and low-carb approaches for serious athletes are rarely long-term solutions and they can seriously hurt your health. But if you're in a phase of training that requires fewer calories or total carbs, yet you want to power through high-intensity workouts, purposeful nutrient timing can bring you the best of both worlds. Such blocks of training are typically found in the off-season, weeks of low mileage or low intensity.

When you are cutting calories and carbs, practicing nutrient timing allows you to stage your fuel (cutting back in the off-hours is preferable to cutting back in the hours surrounding a workout) so you have adequate carb stores on board, along with plenty of extra protein. There's a strong chance this extra protein will be partially utilized as fuel, and you don't want to leave your muscles and amino acid pool deficient in this vital nutrient.

Remember that for performance and health, significant limiting of intake must be temporary. You should return to optimal and adequate fueling when you are looking for high performance or are in a demanding block of training.

Fueling Up for Early Morning Exercise

Ideally, you've primed your body to tackle early morning workouts or practices by prioritizing quality fuel the evening before. This means consuming an adequate meal that's not overwhelmingly large and one which contains all three macronutrients. (Those with a sensitive stomach should aim for low to moderate fat and fiber.) You'll have time to digest and absorb this fuel overnight, and with a primed tank, you can head confidently into an AM workout. Grab a small 100-to-200-calorie snack to fend off hunger before go-time (again, think carbs from low-fiber grains, energy bars, and sports drinks). This small amount shouldn't trigger a blood glucose spike or a rebound valley. And to make your life easier (read: lower rate of perceived exertion), include a cup of coffee 30 or so minutes before the start.

Pro Tip: *Give yourself time to use the facilities. You'll thank me later.*

Even when your alarm fails to go off in time (I see you hitting snooze for the fifth time), you'll benefit from a small snack consumed during an active warm-up. Stacy Sims explains that in the AM, your cortisol levels are elevated, and exercising soon after waking prompts your body to pump out more cortisol, drawing from stores of progesterone, estrogen, and testosterone. Running on empty has a negative impact on the neuropeptide kisspeptin, a neuropeptide responsible for sex hormones and facets of endocrine and reproductive function. Kisspeptin also plays a significant role in maintaining healthy glucose levels, appetite regulation, and body composition. During early morning "training low" sessions or anytime there's insufficient nutrition on board, particularly carbs, kisspeptin stimulation is markedly reduced, creating the potential for increased appetite, reduced sensitivity to insulin, and increasing levels of the stress hormone cortisol. And to think, all this can be avoided with an energy bar, a banana, and a cup of coffee.

Mid-Workout Fueling

Even when starting the workout primed and totally fueled (right?!), you'll inevitably reach a point where your tank starts to become depleted. Adding fuel mid-workout is the key to keeping your tank near full, but you need to choose the right type of "gas." Choose a source of fuel (looking at you, gels) that does not agree with your gut and you'll be fast-tracked to a pit stop. If you try to gut it out on inadequate fuel, when you finally add more to your tank, it'll take a significant amount of time to get back up to speed. Staying primed requires carbohydrates, fluids, and electrolytes, and the longer and faster you're going, the more gas you'll burn. When conditions are extreme, adding in fluid and electrolytes is a must. So take time to lay out your perfect plan, employing trial and error and recording what works and what doesn't.

HOW THE PROS STAY FUELED

DES LINDEN: To perform well, Linden knows she has to train her gut as well as the rest of her body. She often aims for fluids and electrolytes every 5 kilometers, switching to (caffeinated) gels chased with adequate water over longer distances.

TATYANA MCFADDEN: As an elite wheelchair marathoner, McFadden typically completes a race in under 2 hours, but it's an intense and demanding journey. Frequent mid-race fuel includes Powerade, gels, and chews. With limited opportunities to eat and drink during the race, McFadden has a CamelBak attached to her racing chair: "That way I can drink water and push at the same time."

RYAN HALL: During races, for longer efforts lasting over 90 minutes, Hall would take 6 to 8 ounces of a performance (simple carbs) beverage every 3 miles.

MOLLY SEIDEL: Given the countless uncertainties that can arise on race day, Seidel prefers to play it by ear and adapt to the conditions and fuel intuitively, testing as she goes. During her long runs, carbs are king. She usually starts with a bar before go-time, adding in 50 grams of carb each hour from Maurten gels. Seidel says, "A big shift for me was learning to embrace sugar. Stop listening to 'sugar is bad, sugar is wrong,' and instead time it right. Nothing has been better for my ability to come back for another session. Figuring out what I needed during the race definitely helped my performance. Now I know I need 50 grams of carb an hour, and I personally don't need supplemental electrolytes; I just need 5 ounces of water every 5 kilometers."

JOAN BENOIT SAMUELSON: Nine times out of ten, when Joan begins to feel sluggish, she doesn't turn to gels. Never has. She prefers real food first and knows her situation isn't a lack of carbohydrates. It's fluids: "I'm always aware of hydration, because when I start to feel tired, it's typically due to dehydration rather than actual fatigue."

GRAYSON MURPHY: When out traversing trails and mountains, Grayson notes: "I drink water when I'm thirsty, and generally, my training runs do not go over 2 to 2.5 hours, so I don't really have any fueling or hydration strategies. I carry an Ultimate Direction running pack or handheld [pack] and try to include more food and water than I think I will want in case I end up running for longer than I intended to."

WHEN, WHAT, AND WHY OF MID-WORKOUT FUEL

Type of Workout	Fuel Options	Fuel Timing	Why
SHORT EFFORT, LESS THAN 45 MINUTES: SHAKE-OUT RUNS, STRENGTH TRAINING AND CORE, LIGHT EFFORT TRAINING AND PRACTICES	No fuel needed. Top off the tank with 100 to 200 calories if feeling fatigued.	As needed.	Brief exercise utilizes your stores and the fuel you consumed hours ago. Adding in mid-workout fuel isn't usually necessary. Add it if you feel low on energy, your blood glucose is tanking, or you neglected to prioritize pre-workout fueling.

WHEN, WHAT, AND WHY OF MID-WORKOUT FUEL

Type of Workout	Fuel Options	Fuel Timing	Why
45 TO 75 MINUTES AT HIGH INTENSITY: SPEED WORK, TEMPO RUNS, PRACTICES OF LESS THAN 75 MINUTES	Hydrate with water plus electrolytes. Fuel with easy-to-digest sports drink, gels, chews, real food. Add in a sports drink mouth rinse to stimulate parts of brain and central nervous system to help lower RPE and convince yourself to push harder (and love it).	Sip on fluids throughout. Fuel with 30-plus grams of carbs per hour as needed to maintain pace and intensity.	Hard and fast efforts burn through endogenous fuel stores quickly. And if the conditions are hot or humid, hardworking muscles will require more fluids for cooling plus electrolytes to keep contracting and maintain balance. Fuel with easy-to-digest sports drinks, gels, or chews.
60 TO 150 MINUTES: LONG RUNS, RIDES, SWIMS, OLYMPIC DISTANCE TRIATHLON, MOST START-AND-STOP SPORTS	Hydrate with water plus electrolytes. Fuel with easy-to-digest sports drink, gels, chews, real food.	30 to 60 grams of carb per hour. Pepper in carb grams starting at 30 to 45 minutes and space it out. Increase until energy levels remain strong and steady, gut stays happy.	Supplement what's already on board. Your sport will determine your options plus your access to fuel. For team sports, opportunities to add in fuel are typically limited to halftime or water breaks. Make best use of time-outs; prioritize sports drinks, bars, gels, and chews, or even easy-to-digest solid food.
150 MINUTES PLUS: ULTRAS, ENDURANCE RACES, OVERNIGHT RELAYS, IRON DISTANCE TRIATHLON	Hydrate with water plus electrolytes. Fuel with gels and chews that contain a mix of glucose and fructose.	60 to 90 grams of carb per hour. Build across training occasions, adapting your gut from 30 grams per hour toward 90 grams per hour.	Your gut struggles to process more than 1 gram of carb per minute. Fuel with carb sources made from multiple transporters will help achieve the high rate of oxidation required to fuel long efforts. Fuels containing sources of glucose and fructose (these simple sugars are transported differently) will allow you to up your intake and hit the 90-gram mark without your gut retaliating.

Remember, landing on your perfect fueling plan takes trial, error, and record keeping. Once you find options that work for you, don't deviate. Nothing new on game and race day!

NUTRITION FOR THE LONG, LONG RUN

Before you even download a training plan or hire a coach, your best first step is to run to the grocery store. You're about to go through hundreds of thousands of milligrams of electrolytes, tens of thousands of grams of carbs, protein, and fat, many thousands of ounces of fluids, and a seemingly endless number of calories. Trust me, I did the math. The options listed in the table below are a great place to start.

Pro Tip: When that low fuel light comes on, pay attention. If you try to push through energy depletion, replacing and then building back your stores will be a losing battle. Your system is already taxed to the max, working to maintain physiological processes, fluid balance and hydration, blood sugar levels, and more. Don't risk having to play catch-up. Refuel early and often.

Fuel Source	Carb Content (grams per serving) and Source	Other Nutrients	Timing*	Pro Tips	Cautions
GELS	20–25 grams carb from mixed sources Example: Gu Energy original and Roctane, Maurten 100, PowerBar PowerGel, Honey Stinger, Huma Chia Energy Gel, SiS Isotonic Energy Gels	electrolytes +/- BCAAs +/- caffeine	2 to 3 gels per hour	For best tolerance, consume over the course of a mile (or two) rather than all at once.	Chase with water, never with sports drink.

Fuel Source	Carb Content (grams per serving) and Source	Other Nutrients	Timing*	Pro Tips	Cautions
CHEWS	20–25 grams per serving 5–8 grams per chew Example: Clif Bloks, Jelly Belly Sport Beans, Skratch energy chews, PowerBar PowerGel shots, ProBar Bolt energy chews, Honey Stinger energy chews, Gatorade Prime energy chews	electrolytes +/- BCAAs +/- caffeine	1 to 2 chews every 15 minutes, starting at 30 to 45 minutes	Start with chews, fueling early and often. If chewing and transport is too fatiguing, transition to an alternate source later in event.	Chase with water. Difficult to chew—please don't choke—when highly fatigued (late in a race) or in cold conditions.
BARS AND SOLIDS	15–30 grams per serving Example: Clif Bar, Picky Bar, PowerBar Energize Original, UCAN bar, Honey Stinger Waffles, Skratch Sport Crispy Rice Cake	protein, fat, fiber +/- electrolytes +/- BCAAs +/- vitamins and minerals (inherent or fortified)	Pre-race breakfast, halftime snack, bike segment fueling	Tired of gels and chews? Add in a bar for variety. Perfect choice during the bike. Experiment: some are easier to digest.	Sensitive stomach? Avoid bars high in fiber and fat.
"REAL" FOOD	Design to provide 15 to 30 grams per serving	+/- protein, fat, fiber +/- electrolytes (sodium from a pinch of salt; potassium from dried fruit) +/- vitamins and minerals (inherent or fortified)	Pre-race, halftime snack, bike fueling, ultra-long runs	Avoid tons of fruit-only fuel (fructose isn't well tolerated). Experiment with sources of glucose, dextrose, and sucrose. Try maple syrup, honey, candy, mashed salted sweet potatoes, On-the-Go Energy Bites (see the following page), packets of peanut butter crackers, pretzels, mini PB&J sammies, oatmeal-based baby food pouches.	Practice, practice, practice. Train with a variety until you find food-based fuel that is easy to digest and tolerate and is totally transportable.

Fuel Source	Carb Content (grams per serving) and Source	Other Nutrients	Timing*	Pro Tips	Cautions
SPORTS DRINKS (6 TO 8 PERCENT CARB CONCENTRATION)	20 to 25 grams per 12-ounce serving Example: Gatorade (Endurance, original), Powerade, UCAN Energy	electrolytes +/- BCAAs vitamins and minerals (inherent or fortified) +/- other supplements (creatine, herbals, etc.)	Every "water stop" when relying on for fuel. 16 or more ounces per hour to meet fuel needs	Train with what's on the course and at the same intervals drinks will be available at "water stops." If you don't tolerate it, avoid it on race day and bring your own.	Rely on for fuel, not primarily hydration; full octane sports drinks are too highly concentrated to properly hydrate. Carb sources range from simple sugars to complex starches.
ELECTROLYTE DRINKS (0 TO 3 PERCENT CARB CONCENTRATION)	0 to 4 grams per 12 ounces Example: Nuun Sport/Prime, Pedialyte Sport/Advanced Care, Powerade Power Water, UCAN Hydrate	electrolytes +/- glucose +/- BCAAs +/- vitamins and minerals +/- supplements (creatine, herbals, etc.)	Sip during the workout until hydration needs are met	Great choice for hot and humid conditions or when working to quickly rehydrate.	Sensitive stomach? Avoid "low calorie" beverages containing sugar alcohols and artificial sweeteners.

Mix and match. Determine how many grams per hour you need and then add up your sources. You can stick with one source or vary across the workout or race.

RECIPE: ON-THE-GO ENERGY BITES*

Prep Time: 15 minutes active prep

Yield: 8 servings of 4 to 5 bites each

INGREDIENTS:

½ cup nut butter (peanut, almond, sunflower seed)

¼ cup brown rice syrup

¼ cup honey or maple syrup

1 cup old-fashioned rolled oats

1 tablespoon espresso powder (optional)

¼ cup dried fruit (raisins, cranberries, chopped dates)

DIRECTIONS:

1. In a small microwave-safe bowl, combine nut butter, brown rice syrup, and honey or maple syrup. Microwave on high until mixture begins to bubble, approximately 1 to 2 minutes.

2. In a large mixing bowl, combine remaining ingredients and pour in boiled syrup mixture.

3. Stir until thoroughly combined.

4. Cover mixture and chill 1 to 2 hours. Chilling makes mixture easier to handle.

5. Remove from refrigerator and roll into small bites, using about 1 tablespoon ingredients per bite.

6. Divide into 8 individual servings and freeze, using individual snack-size bags, 4 to 5 energy bites per bag.

7. Before a long run, ride, or competition, remove one bag from the freezer and allow to thaw before consuming.

Nutrition Facts per serving (recipe makes 8 servings): 220 calories, 32 g carb, 5 g protein, 8 g fat

Pro Tip: Fuel like the pros . . . or don't. Many elites have nutrition down to a concrete science, but Molly Seidel notes that you'd be surprised by the number who are totally winging it: "I think the thing that people are most surprised by when they talk to me is that I don't have a preset nutrition plan and instead figure out my marathon fueling as I go. I'm generally more loosey-goosey than a lot of marathoners, but perhaps it's because I need to be with my history. For me, intuitively fueling throughout feels better because you simply don't know what race day is going to hand you. You don't know if you're going to drop a bottle or miss a table, so I prefer to be prepared for anything. Everyone has their own approach, but for me, I say take the conditions that you got and just roll with it."

CRITICAL RECOVERY

You know that tired feeling you get after walking up three flights of steps on your way to class? Those leaden legs you get after an intense strength session? The right post-workout fuel can prevent that. The final critical stage of nutrition timing, appropriately referred to as nutritional recovery, serves to replenish run-down nutrient stores, repair and rebuild spent tissue, and reduce stressors so you can fight inflammation and soreness. Here's how to recover from today's workout so you can be primed for tomorrow's, and (most important) avoid that ego-crushing out-of-breath feeling at the top of the stairs.

The Intricacies of Nutritional Recovery

It's amazing how powerful the right nutritional recovery can be. This tool is akin to pre-workout and mid-workout fuel in that you might not realize its true worth until you do it incorrectly. Done *correctly*, nutritional recovery rehydrates and replenishes plasma stores, restocks muscle glycogen stores, and repairs tired and tattered muscles while also preventing further breakdown. All these processes take place via supply of fluids, carbohydrates, and protein, respectively, all consumed in the hours post-workout.

The fitter you are, the smaller your window of recovery and the quicker your nutritional recovery must occur. Clinical studies point to a recovery window—a period when you're metabolically inclined to efficiently absorb and put nutrients to work—as occurring within an hour post-workout coupled with an enhanced sensitivity to fuel (especially protein) in the 24 hours post-workout. As their training demands a lot from their body, elites tend to refuel ASAP. Find their top choices at the end of this section.

Restock and Refuel

Within 60 minutes of finishing a workout, begin rebuilding with 15 to 30 grams of protein and add 0.5 grams of carbohydrate per pound to restock glycogen stores. Bump this up to 30-plus grams of protein during the high hormone phase.

The type of protein you consume here matters. High-quality proteins supplying more than 10 grams of essential amino acids (EAAs) are needed to support training adaptations, and additional supply keeps circulating levels well stocked. Find this amount of EAAs, including leucine, which is critical to recovery, in 15 to 30 grams of dairy (common sources of this easy-to-digest-and-absorb protein include fluid milk, yogurt, and whey protein powders). Purposeful intake helps increase strength and supports favorable changes in body composition.

But don't stop there. The exercise-linked enhancement of muscle protein synthesis responds to further intake of protein within the 24-hour period after exercise. Consume additional protein from complete animal sources and mixed plant protein sources at multiple occasions across the day, peppering in 15 to 30 grams of protein every 3 to 5 hours. Adequate protein mends the microscopic damage inflicted by the workout, so if you fear soreness, loss of lean mass (muscle, bone, and organs), and injury, you'd be wise to prioritize protein.

> **Pro Tip:** Protein powders, smoothies, and on-the-go shakes make for quick refreshing recovery, but don't overlook adding in some carefully curated whole foods. They'll help restore a variety of vitamins and minerals lost in sweat and through metabolism.

If you're in a light phase of training that doesn't demand as many high-octane carbs *and* you don't have any workouts planned in the immediate future, you can take your time with glycogen repletion. Consuming carbs over 24 hours rather than immediately post-workout will still restock stores, albeit not as efficiently. This work-around is helpful if you can't stomach much post-workout or you want to wait for mealtime.

Recovery Right Versus Not . . .

What to expect when you don't recover well? Soreness, fatigue, and malaise are common, but Molly Seidel explains it best: "I feel like trash. I physically cannot handle it. If I don't recover right and don't refuel, I tend to get hypoglycemic and even run the risk of passing out." As such, Seidel recovers with a blend of protein and carbs but doesn't obsess: "I don't count grams or macros or calories. It's triggering for someone who's dealt with an eating disorder, so I eat with a very intuitive approach, simply eating to refuel." With the same trial and error and attention paid to her pre-run meals, Seidel has learned what best aids her recovery.

Remember Rehydration

Sweating depletes the body of fluids and electrolytes, and most athletes finish hard workouts and races in a hypohydrated state. When post-workout rehydration is overlooked (a common practice), recovery is hampered *and* the next workout is begun at a deficit, when you are already in a state of dehydration.

Fluids are critical to both health and future performance, so sip—don't chug—water and add in electrolytes (provided by sports supplements or various whole foods) to effectively rehydrate and retain. Sipping slowly will allow for better absorption while avoiding excessive diuresis or urine losses. Electrolytes—primarily sodium and also chloride, potassium, and sometimes magnesium and calcium—can help retain fluids, especially extracellular fluids inclusive of plasma volume. If you're like many athletes who continue some degree of a sweat fest post-workout, effective rehydration may require intakes above and beyond what you lost in sweat and urine. Recover your losses and then some, aiming for up to 125 to 150 percent of your deficit.

Put it into practice: if you take a sweat test and record losses of 1 pound (16 ounces) across the workout, consume 20 to 24 ounces of fluid during your recovery window. Forgot to do a sweat test? There's a work-around: simply sip on fluids (remember to add electrolytes) until your urine is a light straw color. Dark urine and going more than two hours post-workout without a need to pee is an indication you're not drinking enough.

Drink, Not Drunk

When I say *rehydrate,* I'm not talking about adult beverages. Yes, I'm a killjoy. Alcohol, a known diuretic, is banned by some professional and collegiate teams because it hampers recovery, slows reaction time, lowers inhibitions ("yes, I'll take that third helping of wings and fries, please!"), and fills you up, taking the place of nutrient-dense fuel. Most of alcohol's side effects are commonly a factor of excessive intake, but some athletes choose to avoid alcohol altogether while in season.

Yes, plenty of elites occasionally imbibe: Des Linden is a whiskey lover; Deena Kastor enjoys wine; Molly Seidel finds calories and trace micronutrients in beer. But this intake never trumps training, moderation is paramount, and intake isn't frequent. If you simply love the taste but don't want the ill effects, there are plenty of nonalcoholic options from companies like Gruvi and Athletic Brewing. You can also find options from traditional and craft brewers like BrewDog. The downsides to alcohol far outpace the benefits, so during training and racing, grab a nonalcoholic beer if you love the taste or wait until the season is over to cheers with an adult beverage (and in moderation of course).

HOW THE PROS REFUEL AND RECOVER

KARA GOUCHER: Recovery begins with a 15-gram protein shake, sipped slowly to give her body time to absorb the nutrients: "I try to have a meal within an hour and love a good omelet with breakfast potatoes or hash browns."

ALLIE OSTRANDER: Allie mixes a source of electrolytes (Beam Elevate powder) into her post-workout whey protein shake. Electrolytes are key to her feeling optimally recovered and rehydrated.

RYAN HALL: Ryan grabs a protein shake, opting for quick-digesting whey protein for muscle repair and some fat-free candy to get into the system quickly to replace glucose in the muscle.

DEENA KASTOR: Variety and color often matter most to Deena: "After the run today, I made my daughter and me smoothies with banana, cherries, and avocado. Yesterday post-run was a simple breakfast burrito with egg, avocado, and homemade salsa. Tomorrow will be different, but some combination of protein and carbs with added veggies or fruit for vitamins and minerals."

STEPHANIE BRUCE: The co-founder of Picky Bars was so focused on recovery, searching for a 4:1 mix of carbs to protein, that she helped launch an entire brand. She relies on bars for recovery but also includes protein smoothies, prioritizing protein the closer she is to menstruation. Her go-to smoothie blends fresh mint, cacao nibs, and a banana with rice protein, almond milk, and peanut butter.

Shift Your Mindset and Prioritize

Nutritional recovery serves to prevent excessive post-exercise soreness and fatigue, and hastens the amount of time it takes for muscles to repair. The right plate and mindset will make you a stronger, more resilient athlete, so get into the habit of refueling and rehydrating in the off-season, after light workouts, and most definitely after intense and long efforts. This always-on routine will make future workouts more productive and move you one step closer to your goals.

A DEEP DIVE INTO HYDRATION

There's a clear link between improved performance and optimal hydration. When you are properly hydrated, your heart rate, your core temperature, and your rate of perceived exertion will be lower. Finding your way to optimal hydration takes some careful planning, some trial and error, and ultimately an understanding of what's needed—like the right type and quantities of fluids plus essential electrolytes—to implement an optimal hydration plan.

Electrolytes can be found naturally in various foods as well as in supplements. These nutrients include:

SODIUM: Essential for muscle and nerve function and arguably the most important factor for maintaining hydration status. Sodium is the primary electrolyte in extracellular fluid, so as stores of it are depleted, your plasma volume decreases, impacting your blood pressure, your body temperature, and your ability to cool off.

Source: table salt, salty foods (snacks, processed meats, canned vegetables).

CALCIUM: Responsible for bone health and structure, this electrolyte helps with pH balance, muscle contraction, and nerve transmission.

Source: dairy, leafy greens, seafood, tofu, and various foods fortified with calcium.

CHLORIDE: Along with sodium, chloride exists as a major ion in extracellular fluid and aids in nerve transmission.

Source: table salt, salty foods (snacks, processed meats, canned vegetables).

POTASSIUM: This nutrient of concern (meaning we don't consume enough of it) is a major ion in intracellular fluid, working opposite to sodium. Potassium aids nerve impulse transmission, and insufficient intake can lead to muscle cramps (a fluid volume issue).

Source: dairy, fruits, vegetables, coconut water.

MAGNESIUM: Magnesium is critical for bone strength and nerve and heart function. Too little can lead to weakness, muscle pain, and poor cardiac function.

Source: green leafy vegetables, nuts, legumes, whole grains.

Fluids to support hydration should come primarily from water. Teas, coffee, juices, sports drinks, and low-calorie electrolyte beverages and water-rich fruits and vegetables also contribute to your daily needs.

Time It Right

Your goal is to maintain hydration all day, every day, by regularly sipping on water and maintaining a consistently light yellow urine. Euhydration, the state of being properly hydrated, serves to support health and can help fend off intense cravings and appetite.

If you fail to stay hydrated or to replace significant portions of losses from sweat (a mix of fluid plus electrolytes), you will experience a reduction in plasma and blood volume, forcing your system to pull fluids from other areas of your body. You're left with insufficient fluid to cool you, the potential for GI distress, and more viscous blood. When your heart is forced to work harder to pump thickened blood, your heart rate rises, your risk of heatstroke rises, a greater amount of glycogen is required to fuel the power you simply can't tap into, and you enter into a state of altered cognition (read: poor coordination and increasing levels of self-doubt).

It doesn't take much fluid loss to cause impaired performance; just 2 percent of body weight lost can lead to decreased endurance, premature fatigue, and the inability to find another gear at the end of a race or game. These ill effects occur more often and appear more rapidly in hot, humid conditions, but you're not immune to the possibility of dehydration in winter months. Cold weather dehydration is quite common, resulting as dry and windy conditions increase fluid evaporation, changes in body chemistry hinder the drive to drink, and in order to survive the great outdoors, the body shifts fluids from the extremities to the core, ultimately resulting in increased urine production. While the negative effects of dehydration take longer to appear, showing up as a loss of 3 to 5 percent of body weight, the overall impact is just as real as what you experience in the thick of a hot and humid workout.

Put It into Practice

BEFORE: Start exercise properly hydrated by drinking approximately 1 ounce for every 10 pounds of body weight in the 2 to 4 hours before a workout. Your urine should be pale yellow in color. Stop drinking approximately 20 to 30 minutes before go-time, leaving yourself time to use the facilities.

Example: If you weigh 130 pounds, drink approximately 13 ounces of fluid a few hours before practice or competition.

If you run or work out first thing in the morning and can't fit in both fluids and the time needed to digest, it's wise to hydrate before going to bed at night. If you're concerned about your overall hydration status or the intensely hot and humid conditions in which you'll be competing or training, add a bit of salt to pre-workout meals and drinks. Just a pinch will help you retain the fluid you need and will boost your sodium stores.

DURING: It's difficult to give a blanket recommendation of how much to drink, since baseline hydration status varies, sweat rates are personal, phases of the menstrual cycle impact fluid status, and overhydrating can be more dangerous than underhydrating. Monitor your urine color and perform the sweat test on the following page.

Athletes can lose between 10 and 80 ounces of fluid per hour during exercise, depending on factors such as intensity, duration, heat acclimatization, altitude, apparel, weather conditions, and various physiological parameters. Because fluid shifts occur specific to phases of your menstrual cycle, drink to meet your thirst cues during the luteal phase of your menstrual cycle and utilize your sweat test results, mapping out a hydration plan during menstruation and the follicular phase. All in all, limit total body water losses to less than 2 percent. Remember, you can't simply chug water to prevent dehydration. Overhydration can dilute plasma sodium stores and result in hyponatremia, which is dangerous if not deadly. Because you've got a smaller body size and a lower sweat rate than your male counterparts, you're more likely to drink more than you lose in sweat and urine, putting you at a high risk for hyponatremia (blood sodium less than 135 millimoles per liter).

Play it safe by drinking fluids containing adequate electrolytes and by knowing how much sweat you're losing via a sweat test. Perform the test a few times throughout the weeks of your training, making a note of the conditions and phase of your cycle. That way, regardless of the weather on race or game day and no matter what day the event might fall on, you'll know what kind of sweat losses to expect and you'll have a rock-solid plan in place. For most athletes, an intake of 14 to 27 ounces per hour will suffice.

HOW TO DO A SWEAT TEST: This simple test is well worth the effort. Before and after an hour-long workout, record your weight, then calculate the difference between your weight at the start and your weight at the finish (remember, 1 pound equals 16 ounces of fluid). Add in the amount of fluid consumed during the workout. The resultant number is your goal intake of fluids per hour. Your future fluid strategy should come close to replacing these losses so that you avoid shedding more than 2 percent of your body weight, which spells dehydration and poor performance. Don't take it too far; trying to replace every drop of fluid lost and then some is dangerous.

AFTER: Most athletes finish a workout at a fluid deficit, and rehydration in the minutes and hours post-training needs to be a priority. Rehydration effectively replaces the fluid you've lost and enables your body to recover, especially if you're doing two-a-days or have another workout planned within 24 hours. Incorporate water and potassium-rich fruits and vegetables, as well as salty foods.

When Water Won't Suffice

Those who are salty, gritty sweaters and those who finish a workout soaked (losing more than 1.2 liters per hour) should add electrolytes into water or grab a (hypotonic) sports drink that's formulated for quick rehydration. You need fluids and electrolytes for hydration and sports drinks for energy. Some athletes find that a mouth rinse (that is to say, swishing an ounce of sports drink in your mouth for 5 seconds and then spitting it out) helps too.

Olympic marathoner Molly Seidel notes that "when my stomach is upset, and I simply cannot take a gel, I'll grab some sports drink, swish, and spit. I'm not physically getting those sugars and carbs, but I am getting a boost. I don't know if it's just psychological, but it does help. I can't quantify what it triggers, and maybe I'm just tricking my body to keep going, but no matter what, it works." Research on the mouth rinse suggests this practice enhances executive function and exercise performance primarily because the taste of the carbohydrate solution increases cortical response in motivational reward pathways or perhaps via vagus nerve innervation. While the action does not universally improve endurance in a significant manner, there's certainly no harm in adding this approach to your hydration plan. Just don't count on it to meet your fluid needs.

Quick Options for Optimal Hydration, Rehydration, Recovery

UNDER 1 HOUR WORKOUT

8 ounces water + 1 packet Pedialyte

Isotonic beverages don't fuel you, they rehydrate, thanks to fluids and electrolytes being rapidly shuttled from the gut to the surrounding tissues, saving you from a gut bomb. Grab this type of drink during hot, humid workouts, and add it post-workout for rapid recovery from a dehydrated state.

calories 25

protein 0 g

fat 0 g

carbs 6 g

sodium 240 mg

potassium 180 mg

chloride 290 mg

zinc 2 mg

1+ HOUR WORKOUT

16+ ounces water, 16+ ounces 3–6% carbohydrate solution, including high levels of sodium, chloride, potassium, +/- calcium and magnesium

Meet your fluid needs with water or an isotonic beverage, and fuel with sports drink (or other alternate carb source) to keep pushing the pace. If you have high sweat losses or finish a workout covered in salty grit, you've got significant sodium losses; add electrolytes to your water.

calories under 120

protein 0–1 g (some sports drinks add BCAAs)

fat 0 g

carbs 10–28 g

sodium 230–650 mg

potassium 80–200 mg

calcium 0–115 mg

magnesium 0–40 mg

POST-WORKOUT REHYDRATION AND RECOVERY

1–2 scoops whey protein, 1 cup fortified nut milk or dairy milk, 1 cup ice, 1 cup coconut water, 1 pinch table salt, 1 handful leafy greens, 1 banana

This rehydrating smoothie provides fluids and electrolytes while repleting energy stores and jump-starting muscle recovery.

calories 350–400

protein 25–35 g

fat 5 g

carbs 55 g

fiber 6 g

sodium 450 mg

DEAR YOUNGER, HUNGRY ME: GRAYSON MURPHY

When working to navigate technical trails or pushing the pace across single-track, I'm reminded of the incredible skill and talent of professional runner Grayson Murphy, whose many accolades include first-place finishes at the 2019 and 2021 U.S. Mountain Running, World Mountain Running, and XTERRA Trail Run World Championships. A graduate of the University of Utah, Murphy earned a BS in civil engineering and won NCAA all-American honors five times. Her early athletic foundation was built from soccer and speed, and she evolved to understand that different body types and composition work effectively across sports. Not content to simply run, Grayson uses her athletic reach and influence to create a positive impact and passionately advocates for mental health strength and body positivity. She combines such positivity and an entrepreneurial spirit throughout the pages of her *Racin' Grayson Training Log and Planner*.

Dear Younger, Hungry Little Grayson,

You are fifteen and a sophomore in high school now and have grown in so many ways in just a few short years. Something you should be very proud of! I want to write you this letter to let you know that the next ten years will hold some of the greatest challenges and greatest successes of your life. I know that high school has been difficult to navigate thus far and puberty feels like an unwanted burden that you are trying to run away from. Being called a "woman" is something that you despise right now, but twenty-five-year-old Grayson is pretty proud of her body and the woman that she has become, boobs and all. While it is okay to be uncomfortable in your changing body, please try your best to respect it, because you are going to ask a lot from it.

I know that you deal with anxiety and that you have discovered food as a means of feeling like you're in control. I know, it's a lot. I am not going to tell you that the anxiety or the depression completely goes away as you get older. It is still something that twenty-five-year-old Grayson deals with on a nearly daily basis. But you can take satisfaction and feel calm knowing that your mental health toolbox will continue to grow and thrive and you will soon find more healthy outlets for when your life feels out of control, ones that don't revolve around food.

But beware, what starts out as a control issue with food can and will turn into body image issues if you don't confront the problem with great strength, bravery, and the recognition of your own vulnerability. You are not a runner right now (in fact, right now you think cross-country is the silliest sport you can think of) and soccer is your whole life. You should be very proud of the hard work you have put into that sport! But SURPRISE! In a strange turn of events, you will find running in your sophomore year of college and discover an unknown talent and passion for this new sport. Pay special attention to the lessons around body image you are learning right now and remember those when you enter the world of running. Know that you will see in your competitors some of the most sickly- and unhealthy-looking human beings you have ever seen. Stay true to your strengths and always remember to put your health, both mental and physical, above all else.

It is really easy in the sport of running to be tempted to take shortcuts and drop weight quickly just to achieve a fast time. You will see many of your teammates and competitors do it, so why shouldn't you? Well, twenty-five-year-old Grayson (who is now a world champion, by the way) is here to tell *you that the short-lived fame is not worth it. The damage to your health is not worth it. You will have several tough moments when you begin to stray down an unhealthy path in the next few years, so remember to always check in and be honest with yourself on how you are really doing. Be your own arrow and chart your own course toward what physical and mental health looks like for you. And remember that health is individual and can look different for everyone.*

I know that this feels like a lot right now, so if you don't take anything else away from this letter, please just remember that food is your friend and can help you if you let it and that little Grayson deserves to honor and respect her physical and mental health ALWAYS, even if that means going against the grain sometimes.

Love you endlessly,
Older Grayson

THE IMPACT OF MENSTRUATION

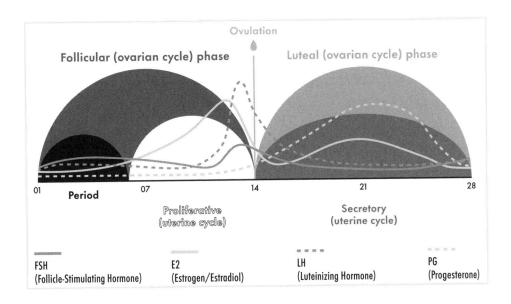

Ovulation

Follicular (ovarian cycle) phase   Luteal (ovarian cycle) phase

01   07   14   21   28

Period

Proliferative
(uterine cycle)

Secretory
(uterine cycle)

FSH
(Follicle-Stimulating Hormone)

E2
(Estrogen/Estradiol)

LH
(Luteinizing Hormone)

PG
(Progesterone)

AN INTRODUCTION TO MENSTRUATION
(OR THINGS YOU NEVER LEARNED IN EIGHTH GRADE)

The menstrual cycle has definite effects on the lifestyle and health of most women, ranging from slight inconvenience to incapacitation. Female athletes acknowledge that it has an impact on performance too. As you read this chapter, you will become aware that the strikingly different perceived rates of exertion you've been experiencing between day-to-day training sessions or competitions are not just in your head. In fact, the ebb and flow of this natural cycle can determine if your performance is on point or if you're even willing to tackle a session at all.

While more and more girls and women are participating in sport, female-centric research in this area is sparse. Exercise science studies have more than twice as many male participants as female. So while specific aspects of performance such as VO_2 max and lactate threshold are known to remain fairly constant throughout the cycle, other factors could vary greatly. Exercise scientists confidently theorize that menstrual hormones have an impact on substrate availability, micronutrient status, thermoregulation, blood plasma volume, fluid balance, and hydration status, but the historic omission of female participation in exercise research has rendered the impact of female physiology on these measurements speculative at best. A clear theoretical and practical understanding of exactly how menstrual cycle phases affect fundamental components of performance and facets of female physiology is lacking.

At present, we've only begun to build a foundation of gender-specific, cycle-specific advice. More studies are on the horizon, but due to the current scarcity of data, each of us must experiment and accept that what works on one day of the month doesn't necessarily work for weeks on end. With this understanding in mind, consider the ensuing advice just a starting point.

Your goal is to better understand *your* cycle, the changes that accompany it, and the potential obstacles and also the benefits it can bring. As you adjust your training and modify your nutrition across phases, take note of what works for *you*.

Go with the Flow: Understanding and Working with Your Menstrual Cycle

The menstrual cycle drives fluctuations in physiology and behavior including mood, metabolism, sleep, and sexual function, as well as growth and development. These factors affect most bodily systems, including integrations with the endocrine system so that the menstrual cycle (as well as your lifestyle, diet, and training routines) consequently impacts glucose metabolism and fuel availability.

The multiple phases of the menstrual cycle—menstruation itself, the follicular phase, ovulation, the luteal, premenstrual phase—each have a unique impact on female physiology. They present unique training and nutrition considerations to attenuate the hormonal flux that can otherwise impact performance.

The average length of the menstrual cycle is 28 days, but outliers beyond the range of 25 to 30 days are common. Most of these irregularities show up around the edges of reproductive life. Regardless of the length of your personal cycle, the duration of the luteal phase is relatively constant, lasting some 14 days. The variability of the cycle typically results from the length of the follicular phase. Yes, there may be average cycle lengths, but avoid thinking of these as normal. There is no normal length of the cycle, no normal response to the effects of the cycle, and no normal impact on metabolism or performance.

Phase 1. Menstruation

WHAT'S GOING ON: Your cycle starts with the shedding of your uterine lining, which lasts approximately 3 to 7 days. Menstruation begins when an unfertilized egg stimulates a drop in hormone levels of estrogen and progesterone.

WHAT YOU'LL NOTICE: You've now entered the *low hormone* phase, during which your hormonal profile is most like your male counterparts.

Your core temperature is lower, you are more easily able to access carbs to hit high intensities, and your mood and power are improved. Your central nervous system (CNS) doesn't fatigue as quickly, and neither do you. You're also more likely to experience uterine cramping and gastrointestinal distress. Heavy periods increase the risk of iron deficiency anemia if your body is not able to increase iron absorption to outpace the rate of loss.

TRAINING STRATEGY: Despite the fact that menstruation poses inconveniences, now is the perfect time to push your limits on speed, endurance, and power.

FUELING STRATEGY: To attenuate common GI symptoms such as diarrhea, nausea, and cramping, Stacy Sims recommends supplementing with magnesium, omega-3 fatty acids, and a low-dose baby aspirin in the week preceding menstruation. Fuel with easy-to-tolerate, GI-friendly foods. If GI upset occurs, replace losses with beverages containing electrolytes, adding in extra potassium and zinc if vomiting occurs. If you are deemed anemic (check with your doctor first or have a lab draw and review your results with a provider like InsideTracker), add in an iron supplement to offset losses.

Pro Tip: Fuel utilization changes across the cycle. Research suggests that the different hormones released during the cycle appear to impact how your body responds to food, energy, and stressors and to influence how your body handles glucose. Thus the reliance on glucose (carbs) and fat for energy production at rest and during training ebbs and flows across the month.

Phase 2. The Follicular Phase

WHAT'S GOING ON: This phase spans the days between the first day of your period and ovulation. This is still a low hormone phase, but as you near ovulation, there is a noticeable increase in estrogen.

WHAT YOU'LL NOTICE: Across this low hormone phase, you continue to experience higher energy levels and have a decreased sensitivity to insulin, which effectively increases your access to blood glucose.

TRAINING STRATEGY: Take full advantage of your peaking energy levels and ability to utilize carbs for fuel; opt for workouts that make you break a serious sweat. Try high-intensity interval training (HIIT) sessions or spinning classes. If you are looking to gain strength (and who isn't?), now is the time to take action; research suggests effective improvements in strength and greater production of force are possible during these days. Do proceed with some caution, however; the rise in estrogen levels as you approach ovulation can increase your risk of injury, so it is important to always listen to your body.

FUELING STRATEGY: Stay hydrated. Follow your usual hydration strategy of meeting fluid losses with fluid replacement. Studies suggest that a sports drink (offering some 55 calories per an 8-ounce serving from carbs along with electrolytes) consumed across the workout (start with ½ ounce per 10 pounds of body weight every 20 minutes) can help improve performance. Math not your thing? Other studies suggest 10 ounces of sports drink every 5 kilometers does the trick. Pro athletes often fall within these two recommendations. Remember to refuel quickly, given that the window of recovery is smaller in women than in men, with a quicker return to baseline. Add in 30 grams of protein, choosing sources that are rich in the amino acid leucine.

Phase 3. Ovulation

WHAT'S GOING ON: The ovulation phase occurs when the mature egg from the follicular phase is released from the surface of the ovary. This generally occurs around the middle of the cycle, approximately 13 to 15 days prior to the start of the next period. Your hypothalamus is triggered to release the hormone GnRH (gonadotropin-releasing hormone). GnRH prompts the pituitary gland to increase levels of luteinizing hormone (LH) and follicle-stimulating hormone (FSH), ultimately triggering ovulation. A critical step in ovulation is the drastic rise in levels of LH. During times of low energy availability and intense training, it is possible to have a cycle in which LH is not significantly increased; thus an egg is not released. This is known as an anovulatory cycle.

WHAT YOU'LL NOTICE: Hormones begin to rise following ovulation, impacting nearly every system in the body, from the luteal phase until menstruation begins again.

Pro Tip: You can track levels of LH and FSH. If you're experiencing cycle irregularities, having difficulty conceiving, or approaching perimenopause, ask your ob-gyn to order lab tests so you can both have insights into what's going on. These two hormones are critical to stimulating an egg to be released, and an anovulatory cycle commonly results from lacking an LH surge. LH levels are tied to several factors, but one you can control is energy availability. Athletes with low energy availability or RED-S are likely to have a decreased LH pulse with an insufficient surge for egg drop. Know your baseline and then work to improve your nutrient intake and energy availability to relax stress on the endocrine system.

TRAINING STRATEGY: Mild side effects such as pain, cramping, nausea, or headaches may hamper your training, but these effects are typically transient. There's a strong possibility that your performance won't be affected during this time. You're shifting from the efficient use of carbs, where you were able to hit high levels of intensity, speed, and strength, to the employment of more fat as fuel, supporting aerobic and endurance capabilities.

FUELING STRATEGY: Fat becomes a preferred fuel, so if racing and competition are on your calendar, hit your desired higher intensities by adding exogenous carbs early and often. Start adding these carbs during warm-up and continue using them intermittently across the workout. Concentrate on drinking when you're thirsty instead of following a set plan so you can prevent dangerously diluting your sodium stores.

Phase 4. The Luteal Phase

WHAT'S GOING ON: You've entered the high hormone phase, an approximately 14-day phase following ovulation and lasting until the start of your next period. Increases in estrogen may make your body more efficient at burning body fat due to an increase in insulin sensitivity, but the increase in progesterone inhibits estrogen and causes a decrease in its sensitivity. This makes the effect of this phase on your metabolism uncertain and difficult to predict.

WHAT YOU'LL NOTICE: If you're trying to push threshold or above, you're likely to fatigue faster. Estrogen shifts fluid out of blood and into other spaces, forcing a drop in plasma volume, which impacts muscle contraction and ultimately leaves less fluid available for sweating. High levels of catabolic progesterone prevent the building of muscle, negatively impact recovery, and drive core temperature up. Overall, you'll notice declines in your time to fatigue and ability to withstand heat.

TRAINING STRATEGY: Now is the time for endurance and aerobic training. You're working harder during this phase; your power drops significantly because you can't access carbs. Factors that affect your rate of perceived exertion (higher core temp, more central nervous system fatigue, less fuel available) are significant and obvious. So less HIIT, more marathon miles, please.

FUELING STRATEGY: Lower levels of circulating leptin, a hormone that decreases hunger, may increase hunger and appetite. Eat mindfully as usual, but do keep moderation in mind.

Elevated estrogen drives a greater reliance on fat along with a limited access to carbs. Some studies suggest this is a detriment to performance, as impaired carb metabolism means an inability to hit high intensities. Conversely, other studies suggest improved fat oxidation and the related preservation of muscle glycogen, increasing your endurance. In other words, the jury is still out!

Enhance fat oxidation by adding in caffeine (3 milligrams per kilogram) and attenuate your inability to hit high intensities by increasing your levels of circulating glucose. Do this by adding in more carbohydrate per hour (aim for up to 0.5 grams per pound per hour, depending on tolerance). If you're in the high hormone phase at the same time your calendar calls for carb loading in preparation for race day, increase your intake above and beyond your usual carb load. Both approaches supply extra carb and will provide access to quick fuel and keep blood glucose levels steady.

> **Pro Tip:** *To see how your blood glucose is impacted by your cycle and whether it's primed to perform, consider adding a continuous glucose monitoring system. You'll be able to track how your body responds to fuel sources across your cycle and be equipped to map out your personal fueling plan.*

As plasma volume drops, fight back by adding in high-sodium foods and fluids, effectively increasing fluid and sodium to expand plasma stores. Drink to thirst, hydrate with a mix of water and electrolytes, and keep the concentration of carbs in your drinks to less than 3 percent. Due to the potential for a reduction in gut permeability in this phase, you'll likely find that high-octane, overly concentrated sports drinks lead to GI distress.

Post-workout, prioritize recovery, as progesterone is catabolic and increases muscle breakdown while thwarting recovery. Consume 30 grams of protein within 30 minutes of finishing the workout. Increase your protein if you're not yet hitting intakes of 1 gram per pound.

Phase 5. The Premenstrual Phase

WHAT'S GOING ON: During the last 6 days of the luteal phase, you'll experience a drastic drop from formerly high levels of estrogen and progesterone. Stress hormone levels (cortisol) and testosterone tend to increase, prompting menstruation and the restart of the cycle.

WHAT YOU'LL NOTICE: A significant rise and fluctuation in hormone levels are responsible for many of the common symptoms associated with premenstrual syndrome: mood changes, headaches, increase in core temperature, acne, fatigue, bloating, and breast tenderness.

TRAINING STRATEGY: Be aware of decreased reaction time and reduced dexterity and neuromuscular coordination if your sport relies on these critical skills. Increased fatigue is common. Fight back by increasing energy availability (that is to say, nutrient timing strategies) during your training. Prioritize rest and recovery especially during times of heavy training, as you may have trouble sleeping because of fluctuating hormone levels.

FUELING STRATEGY: Prioritize carbs before and after training. Supplement with 30 to 40 milligrams of zinc (the upper limit). Zinc deficiency can be linked to fatigue, plus this mineral is a key player in many of the physiological changes that occur immediately prior to your period. Pre-load with 15 grams of protein plus 40 to 50 grams of carb in the hours preceding a long, endurance-specific workout. Add in BCAAs before training or in the early stages of a workout to proactively recover and work against the more negative impacts of estrogen and progesterone.

Compensate for higher core temp and shifts in fluid status by pre-loading hydration, especially when conditions are hot and humid. Add high-sodium foods and soups to your plate, and bring along a beverage that includes sodium to avoid your increased risk of hyponatremia.

Up your overall protein intake throughout the day to lessen the catabolic impact of progesterone and thus reduce the losses of lean muscle mass during this high hormone phase. Find foods that sit well on your stomach, as fluctuating hormone levels often produce lower GI issues. If these impair your ability to fuel properly before a long and taxing workout, prioritize adequate fuel the day before, giving yourself time to digest and absorb.

Clearly, the menstrual cycle is a natural phase that, yes, is sometimes unreliable and is often an inconvenience, but it needn't be a hindrance to performance. Implement tweaks to your training plan, strategize with phase-specific nutrition, and shift your mindset to rise to the occasion no matter the day of the month. You might not be able to control your physiology, but that doesn't mean you have to throw in the towel for days on end across every month.

WHEN YOUR CYCLE GOES AWRY: WHAT'S A GIRL TO DO?

As I pointed out earlier, there is no normal cycle length, but what if your personal cycle is really out of sorts? What if menstruation fails to arrive every 28 days or at all? Losing your period is not okay. The suggestions that you're finally fit enough once you lose your period or that such a loss, termed amenorrhea, will lead to performance improvements are completely erroneous and exacerbate the incidence of amenorrhea, which is commonly underreported and likely impacts as many as 50 percent of female athletes. Amenorrhea typically results from stressors like intense exercise and overtraining, inadequate nutritional support, extreme weight loss, and illness. It's a warning that if something doesn't change, you're about to break.

Warning Flags: Primary and Secondary Amenorrhea

Primary amenorrhea is defined as the absence of menses at age fifteen. There are many genetic and anatomical reasons that a young woman can be older than fifteen and still without a period. The condition results from an immature endocrine system that fails to signal the start of a cycle. Primary amenorrhea in young athletes is often due to energy missteps or not enough fuel intake.

In secondary amenorrhea, menses occur but later disappear. This condition typically develops during the late teens and early twenties. It can result from heavy training loads, low energy availability, and even poor nutrient timing.

Athletes are at high risk when they neglect to consume adequate fuel to meet their baseline resting metabolic rate needs. This lack of calories alters hormone status, forcing the body to down-regulate, opting for survival rather than reproduction. An LH surge will be absent or insufficient, leading to an anovulatory cycle or potentially no cycle. Menstrual cycle dysfunction isn't a badge of honor; it's a warning sign that energy intake isn't matching training demands.

Bringing Back the Period: What Can Be Done?

Supplying the right amounts of the right nutrients at the right time can help. Strategic nutrient timing assures the body that nutrients are coming on board to support the upcoming stress. Recovery fuel begins the restocking and repair process while preventing your body from lingering too long in a pro-inflammatory, stressed-out breakdown state post-exercise.

If you chronically underfuel plus skip nutritional recovery, breakdown continues, and your brain gets the message that the stress is here to stay. In some situations, this high-risk state continues because even though you might effectively take in enough energy throughout the day, consistent misses during the post-workout recovery window cause the signals to get crossed.

To keep regular cycles, you must fuel appropriately. Adequate fuel that supports menstruation also facilitates training adaptations. If you can't stop the breakdown, your body will not be prompted to fully recover from the stress endured and therefore won't adapt or grow stronger. You may be working out, but you're not working out effectively.

Taking Action to Bring Back Your Period and Health

In order to regain your period, your energy balance must be restored. Shifting to a more sedentary lifestyle could work. You'll experience less physical and metabolic stress. Emotional stress is a whole nother ball game. Taking a break from extreme exercise is often the first recommendation of many health care practitioners, who are sensibly focused on the long-term health implications of amenorrhea and RED-S.

Conversely, some coaches and trainers narrowly focused on performance and winning will prioritize training at all costs. Admittedly, sometimes going off the grid when a contract or scholarship is on the line is not realistic. As a compromise, such experts may simply recommend training modifications and hope that menstruation returns.

Many of us are not content to just sit still and wait until our period eventually returns.

Another option is to do fewer highly depleting cardio workouts and turn to strength training, which demands less fuel and helps build lean mass while providing a stress release. Make changes to nutrition too. Do no more workouts in a fasted state, which signals the brain to shift toward a starvation mode and creates a perfect storm of metabolic and endocrine dysfunction. Dump the low-carb plans; you need to boost energy intake and availability in and around training in order to avoid a catabolic state. Carbs on board will help stimulate kisspeptin, helping to "wake up" luteinizing hormone and thus support that LH pulse so critical to stimulating ovulation.

How much does it take to fix the low energy availability that is driving menstrual dysfunction? The solution varies from athlete to athlete, with many practitioners prescribing upwards of 1,000 calories periodized around training (split before, during, and after). This may seem like a lot of fuel, but given the level of deficiency, it's critical. Divided in and around a workout, this calorie intake is manageable, supports body composition goals, and buttresses the most important outcome: your long-term health.

So if you've lost your period, you need to go find it—now. Seek a compromise in training and nutrition that you can live with so you can finally live fully. With the right approach in place, your period will return, RED-S will fade, and you will experience better health, energy, and performance.

FIRESIDE CHAT:
WHEN EATING GOES AWRY

Athletes often at one point or another restrict their food intake or engage in excessive physical activity. Their reasons range from manipulating their body composition for health or for improved performance to feeling better in their own skin to chasing an unreasonable level of thinness. Taken to extremes, restricted eating can evolve into disordered eating and potentially a clinical eating disorder. But before you start worrying that trying to change your body composition will inevitably result in a mental health battle or that low energy availability (LEA) will result from purposeful restriction, be assured that this is not always the case. LEA may occur because of heavy training schedules, decreased hunger, poor knowledge of nutrition, or even reduced access to food throughout the day.

Regardless of the reason(s), when an athlete tries to operate with an ongoing energy deficit, the body responds physiologically by trying to conserve energy. The signs and symptoms of this are similar to those observed in malnourished or even starving populations: lower resting metabolism, low body temperature, low body weight, alterations in metabolic hormone profile, poor bone integrity, severe nutrient deficiencies, and so forth. These same signs and symptoms are also common to certain clinical eating disorders.

LOW ENERGY AVAILABILITY AND
RELATIVE ENERGY DEFICIENCY IN SPORT

Problems begin to emerge when an athlete, intentionally or unintentionally, fails again and again to consume enough calories to meet the energy demands of sport plus the energy required to support health, general activity, growth, and training adaptations.

Low energy availability (LEA) occurs when there is a mismatch between what you're eating (energy intake) and the energy you expend during exercise, ultimately leaving you with inadequate energy to support the functions required by the body to maintain optimal health and performance.

A chronic and severely insufficient intake causes a state of low energy availability known as relative energy deficiency in sport (RED-S). By definition, the syndrome of RED-S refers to "impaired physiological functioning caused by relative energy deficiency and includes, but is not limited to, impairments of metabolic rate, menstrual function, bone health, immunity, protein synthesis and cardiovascular health." LEA underpins RED-S. Similar to disordered eating, RED-S does not begin or exist at one specific point. Instead, it exists on a spectrum ranging from skipping meals occasionally to severely restricting calories and engaging in pathological weight control behaviors similar to those of individuals diagnosed with clinical eating disorders.

Part of RED-S is a triangulation of symptoms formerly known as the female athlete triad (a term that is still commonly used today). Historically, the female athlete triad consists of three interrelated conditions that, in their most severe form, include the state of low energy availability, a loss or disruption in menstrual cycle, and impaired bone health. Since there are more than three factors impacted by insufficient energy availability and because such a range of factors is not limited just to women, the term itself was not as encompassing as necessary.

With the goal of protecting athletes' health, the International Olympic Committee (IOC) developed two RED-S models illustrating the many health and performance consequences associated with RED-S.

Pro Tip: *Rachel Hannah, a sports dietitian and elite Canadian endurance athlete, warns that not all signs and symptoms of RED-S are obvious. "Just because you have your period doesn't mean that you are properly fueled. Poor sleep, difficult time recovering, and other (seemingly insignificant) symptoms can indicate underfueling and LEA."*

Health Consequences of Relative Energy Deficiency in Sport (RED-S)

- Psychological consequences (either preceding RED-S or the result of RED-S)
- Dysfunction in immune system, GI system, menstrual health, metabolism, hematology, endocrine system
- Cardiovascular concerns
- Growth and development delay and hindrance
- Impaired bone health

Performance Consequences of Relative Energy Deficiency in Sport (RED-S)

- Decreases in endurance performance, strength, responses to training, coordination, concentration, glycogen stores
- Increases in injury risk, impaired judgment, poor mood and irritability, depression

LISTEN TO YOUR BODY, AND THAT TINY VOICE INSIDE

This is not a book about eating disorders. Instead, it is about fueling performance and health, a journey to build a better relationship with food. But the two areas may intersect in dark ways at one point or another as a result of offhand comments, negative commentary,

Pro Tip: *Clinical eating disorders may be more common than you might believe, but the incidence of LEA, RED-S, and the types of behaviors that could evolve into dark days far surpasses diagnosed conditions. In a survey assessing the eating behaviors (binging, purging, restrictive food choices), exercise behaviors, and attitudes toward body image and weight reduction of Division III female athletes, nearly 30 percent exhibited risky eating behaviors that could develop into eating disorders. And over 25 percent responded in a way that suggested they were at risk. Nearly 6 percent of the female athletes who completed the survey had a clinical eating disorder.*

genetic predisposition, environment, or the linking of self-worth to weight and nutrition. It's time to bring these issues out into the open and talk about them.

News coverage may prompt you to believe that eating disorders are quick, transient, and manageable, but they are anything but. Poor relationships with food and self, disordered eating, and eating disorders are insidious, persistent, and complex, and once they are entrenched, they grow only more powerful the longer they persist. They rebel against reason. They ignore body signals. They reinforce negative symptoms and behaviors until disordered eating is normalized.

Comments on the appearance of someone else, even when said in an effort to compliment or motivate the individual, can add fuel to a dangerous flame. And the flame is fanned as food intake and habits and weight transition from healthy to dangerous. Eventually you're dealing with an out-of-control wildfire.

Who's at Risk?

The answer to the question of who is most at risk of disordered eating and eating disorders is fairly straightforward and reflected in the mirror. It's you. And me. And those participating in aesthetically judged, gravitational, and weight-class sports. Really no sport is exempt. It's most often the very same population deemed too fragile, complex, or delicate to study: adolescents, teens, young adults. And while the condition develops most often in women, men are not immune. When asked about the state of sport and body positivity, Ryan Hall confided: "Let's just say I am glad conversations are happening. There weren't a lot of guys talking about eating disorders when I was coming up. The issue is pretty silent on the guys' side, but that isn't because it isn't happening pretty often. This is a real issue for both genders." Hall's statement is spot-on: a staggering 20 million American women and 10 million American men are likely to be afflicted by an ED at some point in their lives. This is equivalent to 9 percent of the U.S. population, a statistic that mirrors the global incidence of eating disorders, but athletes far outpace these rates. Depending on the sport as well as the study cited, athletes are more likely to experience eating disorders, with the prevalence ranging up to 19 percent in male athletes and 6 to 45 percent in female athletes.

> **Pro Tip:** If you're glancing over this chapter, thinking broken relationships with food have not, will not ever affect you, you're wrong. As an athlete you're bound to see them in your own tribe, may be called on to help a teammate or friend, and may even wage your own battle with them.

The Warning Signs

You've got an inkling that your feelings around food and self may have taken a wrong turn. Here is a short list of some of the common warning signs as well as risk factors and consequences surrounding clinical eating disorders. Researchers investigating factors that facilitated student-athletes' recovery from their eating disorder found the desire to be healthy enough to perform in sport to be the most powerful motivation.

Physical/Medical Signs and Symptoms	Psychological/Behavioral Signs and Symptoms
➤ Amenorrhea ➤ Hypothermia (cold intolerance) ➤ Noticeable fluctuations in weight, often with significant weight loss ➤ Gastrointestinal complaints ➤ Dizziness upon standing ➤ Difficulty concentrating, sleeping ➤ Signs and symptoms surrounding dental, skin, hair, and nail health ➤ Bone injury—bone stress, fractures, breaks ➤ Hormone dysfunction (including dysregulated menstrual cycle, libido, and erectile function) ➤ Frequent illness, lethargy	➤ Anxiety and/or depression ➤ Weight loss, dieting, and control of food are priorities and may evolve into a debilitating preoccupation ➤ Claims of "feeling fat" despite being thin ➤ Excessive exercise ➤ Difficulty concentrating ➤ Use of laxatives and diet pills ➤ Food rituals and restrictive eating; reducing/eliminating food groups and macronutrients; reducing overall energy intake; counting, measuring, weighing food obsessively ➤ Social withdrawal, including avoidance of food-related social activities ➤ Frequent dieting, body checking ➤ Extreme mood swings and irritability ➤ Bathroom visits after meals
Health Consequences	**Risk Factors in the Sport Environment**
➤ Purging behaviors that cause electrolyte imbalances with possible irregular heartbeats and heart failure ➤ Stress fractures (and overuse injuries) ➤ Premature osteoporosis ➤ Peptic ulcers, pancreatitis, and gastric rupture ➤ Dental and gum problems ➤ Muscle cramps, weakness or fatigue	➤ Sport body stereotypes and belief that losing weight will increase performance ➤ Pressure (real or perceived) from coaches and others to lose weight ➤ Observed eating and exercise behaviors of teammates and competitors ➤ Revealing uniforms ➤ Presumption of health based on performance

Performance Consequences

➤ Protein burned as fuel: Restricting carbohydrates can lead to glycogen depletion, forcing the body to compensate by burning protein and robbing muscle, thus increasing the risk of muscle injury and weakness.

➤ Declining VO_2 max: Low energy can negatively affect VO_2 max and top speed, intensities.

➤ Cognitive and mood consequences: The athlete is malnourished, dehydrated, depressed, anxious, and obsessed with eating, food, and weight. This affects her or his ability to concentrate as well as to manage emotions.

➤ Performance-impacting dehydration, caused by vomiting, restriction, and excessive exercise.

➤ Poor bone health: Low energy availability can disrupt hormones, resulting in compromised bone density and increased risk of bone injuries, including stress fractures.

THE WHY *OF EATING DISORDERS*

There are countless reasons why eating can go awry: genetics and biology, family history, other mental health disorders (such as anxiety disorder, depression, obsessive-compulsive disorder), general psychological health, trauma (neglect, abuse and assault, teasing, and bullying), and stress can all contribute.

These many and varied factors explain why eating disorders are ironically not about food. Clinicians explain that the pervasive nature of struggles with mental health means few individuals are totally immune to the risk. If you're feeling desperately alone or like you have to fight in secret, don't.

A desire for control accompanied by a loss of control is a common theme underlying many eating disorders. Grayson Murphy's struggles initially stemmed from stress and a fixation on food—one factor she had within her control. She grew up in a household where her family bonded over meals, her mom was an amazing cook, and there was no negativity surrounding eating. Rather, her struggles were sparked by a stressful incident. After Murphy didn't make the varsity soccer team, making the junior varsity as a freshman instead, she turned to restriction as a form of self-induced punishment. But when others mentioned how small she was, restriction morphed into body image struggles, further exacerbated by comments suggesting a petite look was desirable. Driven, she continued to work toward making the varsity team and succeeded in her quest, but the fact that she was still restricting her eating meant she wasn't fueled to tackle the challenge of competing. What flipped the switch? "I got to a point where sports were threatened to be taken away if I didn't change. Simultaneously, I saw the U.S. women's national team play and realized they were strong. I realized I cared more about soccer than body image."

But while she was encouraged to gain weight—indeed, gaining weight was critical to her success—she notes the process was uncomfortable, and the body size deemed essential for competition wasn't what she was made for. Most of us are naturally predisposed to a specific weight range where health and performance come to life. Training to put on bulk and mass can be as difficult to navigate as training to achieve a racing weight. Either approach should be viewed as a temporary phase so as to not create a foundation for long-term consequences.

Murphy sought a different outlet for sport, turning to running, a sport in which everyone strove to be smaller. "Sometimes races seemed like a different world, with undernourished people everywhere." She still got the same unsolicited comments and even compliments over her small size, but this time she was able to take these in stride. "I had changed my perspective and was farther removed. I could see how sport changes the conversation." But while her mindset remains healthy, Murphy acknowledges the fact that recovery isn't linear. "It's a long process of keeping the switch flipped."

Molly Seidel struggled with an eating disorder while at Notre Dame, her obsessive-compulsive disorder manifesting itself as stringent restriction and excessive exercise. She kept restricting and was even told to lose weight until she broke down, suffering injury after injury. She grimaces when she thinks of being at her lowest, darkest point and worries that other athletes will see images of her winning and think that's the type of body needed to be a runner. She advises: "Success can be so empty. Don't take Instagram and social media and pictures at face value. Everybody is going through stuff. Just because someone is winning doesn't mean they are happy and fulfilled. Just because someone didn't win doesn't mean that they aren't better off in every facet of their life. It doesn't matter where you're finishing as long as you're doing what you need to be doing."

THE BATTLE AT HAND: EATING DISORDER OR DISORDERED EATING?

First, know that if you are concerned about having an eating disorder or disordered eating, ask for help. Don't be embarrassed. Don't feel ashamed. There is absolutely nothing wrong with raising your hand and saying that you think your food and that number on the scale might be taking over your life. If more people spoke up and sooner, there'd be less taboo, less suffering in silence.

Eating disorders are serious mental health illnesses that carry grave consequences. They have the highest mortality rate of any mental illness, and if left unaddressed, they can linger for decades. Clinicians agree that the sooner your thinking begins to change, the better the outcome. Hence we all need to better understand what these illnesses entail—their potential causes and remedies—and how to get help or to be of help to a friend, teammate, or loved one.

How do you know if you or someone you care about is battling disordered eating or an eating disorder? The foundation of an eating disorder is a preoccupation with food, body weight, and body shape that leads to behaviors such as starvation, fasting, binge eating/purging, and excessive exercise. What often starts as curiosity grows into a preoccupation. Those who suffer from these disorders lose control as obsession takes over, becoming a priority over school, social life, family life, relationships, health, and eventually performance.

Disordered eating is a broad term, describing the spectrum from optimized nutrition through to clinical eating disorders. A person's position on this spectrum isn't necessarily fixed; eating patterns and behaviors shift along the spectrum, fluctuating with stages of life, training cycle, chosen sport, even stage of therapy when needed. Athletes are more likely to succumb to disordered eating than to a clinical eating disorder, and they have a higher incidence of both conditions than do nonathletes.

The symptomatology of disordered eating is similar to that of an eating disorder, but disordered eating does not check all the boxes necessary for a clinical diagnosis. Disordered eating may look very much the same as a clinical condition, including short-term or somewhat chronic behaviors like regularly skipping meals, excessively exercising, and binge eating and purging, but it stops short of fully meeting the criteria for an ED.

In need of a little more information in hand before you reach out for aid? See the chart on the following page. For a comparison of the common characteristics of a clinical eating disorder and disordered eating. Remember, it's possible and probable for your relationship with food to change over the course of your athletic career, to be different from season to season or from one phase of training to another. But to prevent a debilitating preoccupation with food, speak up. Reach out as early and as often as you need it. You don't want to move from one end of this spectrum to the other for the rest of your life.

AT A GLANCE:
COMMON CHARACTERISTICS OF EATING DISORDERS AND DISORDERED EATING

Clinical Eating Disorder	Disordered Eating
Clinically significant behaviors used to control weight—restriction, purging, binging—that occur multiple times per week.	Behaviors used to control weight that occur occasionally but not regularly.
Thoughts of food, eating, calories, tracking intake seemingly take over one's waking hours.	Thoughts of food, eating, calorie burn, and so forth do not own every waking hour.
Preoccupation with food, weight, and calorie burn interferes with social life, performance, and flexibility of schedule.	Scheduling, flexibility, ability to eat when, where, whatever remains intact.
Significant dietary restriction often based on a desire to "eat healthy" or avoid foods/food groups/ingredients results in insufficient intake.	A preoccupation with "eating healthy" or "eating clean" may be present, but intake remains sufficient to support health and performance.
Exercise is excessive—beyond that prescribed/recommended by health authorities or coaches, typically for reasons of calorie burn.	Exercise follows a plan prescribed/mandated/recommended by health authorities or coaches. It is not excessive, and while calorie burn may be one factor of focus, it is not a primary reason for exercise.
Meets specific criteria outlined in *DSM-5*.	

Clinical eating disorders are serious health conditions, and as such, they demand careful diagnosis through clinical classification via the *Diagnostic and Statistical Manual of Mental Disorders* (*DSM-5*), followed by individual treatment plans to facilitate recovery. Statistics suggest that most athletes may experience a degree of low energy availability and potentially disordered eating but will not experience such clinical conditions. Anecdotally, eating disorders are likely more prevalent than research might capture and are on an uptick following the COVID-19 pandemic.

There is a degree of overlap across clinical eating disorders, with some signs and symptoms, risk factors, prevalence, and health implications unique to each condition. Resources are available to provide help and support and further explore the ins and outs of common eating disorders. On the following page is a glossary of these conditions. To further understand intricacies of each condition, refer to some of the notes cited in this chapter.

CLINICAL EATING DISORDERS

ANOREXIA NERVOSA (AN): An eating disorder characterized by significant restriction of energy intake relative to requirements; weight loss (or lack of appropriate weight gain across periods of growth during childhood); difficulties maintaining an appropriate body weight for height, age, and stature; an intense fear of gaining weight, even though currently underweight; and in many individuals, a distorted body image. AN involves a significant restriction of calories and the types of foods consumed. Compulsive exercise, purging, laxative use, and/or binge eating may also be present.

BULIMIA NERVOSA (BN): An eating disorder characterized by a cycle of binge eating (consuming an amount of food that is significant over a discrete period of time (e.g., within any 2-hour period)), a feeling of lack of control during the episode, plus recurrent inappropriate compensatory behavior in order to prevent weight gain, such as self-induced vomiting, misuse of laxatives, diuretics, or other medications, fasting, or excessive exercise.

BINGE EATING DISORDER (BED): A severe, life-threatening eating disorder that is clinically and anecdotally the most common eating disorder in the United States. BED is characterized by recurrent episodes of eating large quantities of food (often to the point of great discomfort), a feeling of a loss of control during the binging episode, as well as great distress, disgust, depression following each episode. Inappropriate, unhealthy compensatory measures are not used to counter the binge eating.

ORTHOREXIA NERVOSA: First described in the late 1990s, this condition involves an obsession with proper or "healthful" eating. It is not recognized as a clinical eating disorder by *DMS-5*, but its incidence is on the rise. Significant restriction of the amount and types of foods eaten can result in severe malnutrition. Therapy for orthorexia often mirrors that designed around anorexia nervosa or obsessive-compulsive disorder.

OTHER SPECIFIED FEEDING OR EATING DISORDER (OSFED); PREVIOUSLY REFERRED TO AS EATING DISORDER NOT OTHERWISE SPECIFIED (EDNOS): OSFED refers to a category of serious life-threatening disorders that do not meet the strict diagnostic criteria for AN or BN or BED. Still, a serious eating disorder exists, carrying health implications and requiring intervention.

Health Consequences of Eating Disorders

The human body is an amazingly resilient machine, equipped to cope with disordered eating and eating disorder behaviors, so sometimes the health consequences take time to appear and not all signs and symptoms present.

During the severe and chronic restriction indicative of anorexia nervosa and which accompanies other similar conditions, the body is literally starved of the nutrients it needs to thrive. As a result, reserves are drained, and as the tank nears empty, the body is forced to slow down all its processes to conserve energy. Serious medical consequences arise.

The recurrent binge-and-purge cycles of bulimia nervosa will impact the integrity of bones, skin, teeth, and gums. The entire digestive system can be negatively impacted, leading to electrolyte and chemical imbalances (a common concern across all EDs), affecting the heart and other major organ functions.

The health risks of binge eating disorder are most commonly the same concerns associated with clinical obesity: weight stigma and cyclical weight fluctuations (loss and then gain and so on). It's important to note that BED can be diagnosed at any weight, and the majority of people deemed clinically obese do not have BED.

All clinical eating disorders carry significant and numerous health consequences. Thus the reason for education and early intervention so that long-term health consequences might be avoided. Not all consequences are readily apparent or even seen across clinical labs and markers. Even after a patient has had an eating disorder for a long time, laboratory tests can generally appear perfect even when he or she is at the point of death. But electrolyte imbalances and cardiac arrest can kill without warning.

Fighting the Battle: Start Here

When it comes to battles with ED and DE, progress with blinders on and be selfish about it. Be focused on your goal to build a better relationship with food and self, finding sustenance that builds a better and healthier you, no matter what it takes or what people might think. Put in the work and have the necessary conversations. If you're not in a good place yet, you've got company. Countless high school students, college co-eds, working professionals, moms, dads, and friends are working to navigate a world packed with confusing advice and misinformation or are taking steps down the wrong path. But the goal for all is to return to the brighter road as fast as possible.

The Many Ways to Help a Teammate or Loved One

A full team of medical professionals is required to help someone recover from a clinical eating disorder. These complex and dynamic conditions demand professional help. But you can offer support to a teammate or loved one in many ways.

EDUCATION IS CRITICAL: You're already starting off on the right foot, because the more you know about what your teammate or loved one is going through, the better you can support them. Everyone is different, so don't make assumptions and don't be afraid to ask questions about their individual experience with an eating disorder.

SPEAK UP: If you're worried about a friend, have a critical, albeit uncomfortable conversation. Speak from your own point of view, using terms like "I'm concerned about . . ." or "I've noticed XYZ and I was wondering if we could talk about it?" Don't point fingers or place blame with lines like "You've got me really worried" or "You've got to stop doing XYZ."

OFFER SUPPORT: An important component to recovery is the ability to derive support from a network of people. Remember that oftentimes eating disorders develop as a way to cope with difficult emotions, thoughts, or events. A friend, teammate, or loved one can lend emotional support so that the reliance on the eating disorder becomes less necessary. Many people who live with eating disorders feel high levels of shame, and experience stigma from the outside world. Joining with your loved one in therapy groups, when invited, sends a message of empathy, acceptance, and love that can help them move past those feelings of shame.

WATCH YOUR WORDS: Talking about physical appearance, body size, and weight isn't helpful to someone in the middle of an eating disorder. This goes for both compliments and criticisms.

REMAIN SELF-AWARE: You're here to be supportive, but you don't have to completely overhaul your own life to accommodate the eating disorder. You can reach out to parents, teachers, or professionals who are more likely to be equipped with resources. Set boundaries and remember to protect your own mental health.

DON'T GIVE UP: No matter what, don't give up hope. Sometimes recovery from an eating disorder arrives quickly. Sometimes it takes decades. Sometimes recovery comes and goes. But sustained and permanent recovery from an eating disorder is possible. The road to being fully recovered is neither easy nor always linear, but having support along the way makes the journey a little easier.

Use Your Tools

Across these pages you've likely paused to reflect on your own personal nutrition journey and your future path. Perhaps your trajectory changed for better or worse based on one comment or one person's opinion. Maybe it changed again when you learned food is the substrate for powerful muscle and the source of hydrating nutrients. You are strong enough, brave enough, smart enough. Now go choose your own path.

You've learned to embrace food as a tool to aid performance and health rather than see it just as an obstacle or an annoyance. You're equipped with the knowledge to fuel your health and your performance and, perhaps more important, to resist dark days and poorly lit paths. Hopefully, you've learned how to help others along the way. Yes, your little light can make the difference for someone headed toward dark days and nutritional missteps. Keep it brightly shining.

Remember that knowledge is power. Use yours to help us all move from a place of being misinformed, underfueled, and feeling lost, depleted, and at war with self and sport.

Keep these conversations going. It will take a village to fix universal problems of body criticism and dissatisfaction, fear of food, and eating disorders. We need more data to drive health and performance and expose the intricacies that women experience daily. It's time to uncover the right information and get it into the hands of more young, seasoned, and aspiring female athletes. Let's help others understand they aren't alone in this journey. There's always a light at the end of the tunnel because someone cared enough to show the way.

Dear Younger, Hungry Me,

Let me give you a hug. I know you need one after being told, once again, that you eat too much, that you should start running more because your thighs are getting fat, or that you don't have what it takes to be a professional athlete. Alongside this hug, I'll even let you in on a secret that I uncovered after years of clawing out of dark places and constant battles with the internal voice named Can't. And that is, if you listen to others when they tell you that you aren't good enough or you don't have the body type that fits the image of sport, then you'll start to believe their lies.

If just for one moment, let's ignore the critics and instead consider some advice that doesn't start with the all-too-familiar "Don't take this the wrong way . . ." Advice gleaned over years of hard work, tears, and grit, and stemming from a reflection of what I wish I would have done.

First, there is no one perfect way to fuel body or performance. One day you'll be a sports dietitian, which makes the aforementioned statement a bit ironic, but in truth, every single person is their own experiment, an n of 1. What works for one person doesn't necessarily work for another. Question everything. Through trial and error, you'll discover the types and amounts of food that work—or don't—to fuel and nourish you. Your plate will evolve over time, as will your body, your skills, your passions.

Next, there will be days you feel fat. We all have them. You'll be in the midst of a "sky's the limit" kind of day and suddenly be blindsided by a glance in the mirror. Stop. Don't give this reflection the power to ruin even the smallest fraction of your life. Like the size of your pants or your shoes, the number on the scale is just a number. It has nothing to do with your worth as a person. It's one metric out of many, offering insight to where you are at one moment in time. The more power you give to the mirror or the number on the scale, the stronger it becomes and the weaker you become. Fight back. Stay strong. You are so much more than a number. When you're feeling derailed, read this paragraph again.

Next, you really will be more disappointed by the things that you didn't do than by the ones you did do. So when you compete in a triathlon and finish near the top, accept the invitation to compete with the pros. Don't let your fears hold you back. Instead, learn to swim—for real—and then see what happens when you jump in the deep end.

Next, it's okay to eat. Crazy, right? In the world of nutrition, there's hunger and there's appetite. Hunger is the physiological drive to eat, an innate survival mechanism informing you when the fuel tank runs low and requires a refill. You can replenish the tank with high-quality fuel (always recommended) or with cheap fuel (a sometimes choice), but the tank must have something in it to move forward. Appetite is in your head, but that doesn't mean it's not real. Watch those external cues and think it through before you grasp for a way to cope and numb feelings with food. You can work to silence cravings or respond in healthy ways. But don't totally tune out cravings: there are some wonderfully delicious foods in the world that you'll miss if you're rigidly inflexible. Hunger is invaluable, a fuel gauge to warn you before you hit empty. You will see teammates and friends misusing both tools. Be brave enough to help them if you can. And be brave enough to help that person in the mirror too. Be kind to your own body. After all, you get only one. Listen and respond accordingly to fuel your miles, and when you fall down a rabbit hole, find help. You're going to need to ask more than one person for directions, but keep asking until you find your way back to you.

Finally, don't let the obsession with food or weight swallow years of time. Don't let someone else's insensitivity dampen that bright and shining light you have within you. No one has the right to take away your dreams or cause you pain and rob you of confidence. Work to view food as the fuel you need to chase your passion. Some days are tough, but, my darling, so are you.

ACKNOWLEDGMENTS

This book was made possible because enough women believed it's time for better. Because the powerhouse team at Avery books, especially my gifted editor, Hannah Steigmeyer, believed it was time for a change. This project was brought to life because my amazing agent and friend Eryn Kalavsky believed in this project from the very beginning.

These pages are filled with moving stories and insights because talented athletes and experts felt compelled to make a change. Without the willingness of Tatyana McFadden, Ryan Hall, Deena Kastor, Des Linden, Grayson Murphy, Allie Ostrander, Kara Goucher, Rachel Hannah, Stephanie Bruce, Molly Seidel, and Joan Benoit Samuelson to dig deep and share their personal journeys, this book would simply not have been possible. I'm indebted to you all.

I'm grateful to Jen Van Allen and Rachel Hibbard, who each have a keen eye for edits and an amazing way with words. To Chris Miller, Mary Kate Shea, and others who opened doors and made introductions. To Sarah Sharp, a talented clinician who loves sports nutrition more than I do, if that's remotely possible. Thank you to my confidantes Jenna Bell, Katie Gunderson, Lindsey Gerba, and Jennifer Sharp, who were unfailingly supportive and encouraging across many (many!) months of writing.

Finally, I wrote this book because my dad taught me from an early age that I was strong enough to make a difference and tough enough to do hard things. I wrote it from the sidelines of soccer games and from park benches while my children played. Miller, Hunter, and Piper, every word was written with the hope of creating a better world for you. I wrote this book on evenings and weekends while Judy and Lou, Joan, and Grace Lawless kept my children alive and the house in one piece. I wrote this book in the early hours, at night, and on weekends while my husband, Jason, held down the fort, and kept me on track (or tried to!), supporting me as I did something I love. I'm eternally grateful to each one of you. And finally, I wrote this book inspired by watching my fierce and fearless mom embrace every moment she's given. All that I am or hope to be, I owe to her.

NOTES

MAPPING OUT DAILY ENERGY NEEDS

14 **physical behavior that emanates from an unconscious drive for movement:** Catherine M. Kotz, Claudio E. Perez-Leighton, Jennifer A. Teske, and Charles J. Billington. "Spontaneous Physical Activity Defends Against Obesity." *Current Obesity Reports* 6, no. 4 (2017): 362–70. doi: 10.1007/s13679-017-0288-1.

14 **energy expended for everything we do that is not sleeping, eating, or sports-like exercise:** James A. Levine. "Non-Exercise Activity Thermogenesis (NEAT)." *Best Practice & Research Clinical Endocrinology & Metabolism* 16, no. 4 (2002): 679–702. doi: 10.1053/beem.2002.0227.

15 **The luteal phase of the menstrual cycle:** Melissa J. Benton, Andrea M. Hutchins, and J. Jay Dawes. "Effect of Menstrual Cycle on Resting Metabolism: A Systematic Review and Meta-Analysis." *PLoS One* 15, no. 7 (2020): e0236025. doi: 10.1371/journal.pone.0236025.

17 **BMIs categorized as underweight:** J. Lim and H. S. Park. 2016. "Relationship Between Underweight, Bone Mineral Density and Skeletal Muscle Index in Premenopausal Korean Women." *International Journal of Clinical Practice* 70, no. 6 (2016): 462–68. doi: 10.1111/ijcp.12801.

18 **BMI is classified into:** Centers for Disease Control and Prevention. "Defining Adult Overweight & Obesity." *https://www.cdc.gov/obesity/adult/defining.html;* accessed July 30, 2021.

18 **IBW, much like BMI, should be taken with a grain of salt:** Courtney M. Peterson, Diana M. Thomas, George L. Blackburn, and Steven B. Heymsfield. "Universal Equation for Estimating Ideal Body Weight and Body Weight at Any BMI." *American Journal of Clinical Nutrition* 103, no. 5 (2016): 1197–203. doi: 10.3945/ajcn.115.121178.

18 **Finally, researchers have analyzed:** Bhumika Shah, Kathryn Sucher, and Claire B. Hollenbeck. "Comparison of Ideal Body Weight Equations and Published Height-Weight Tables with Body Mass Index Tables for Healthy Adults in the United States." *Nutrition in Clinical Practice* no. 3 (2006): 312–19. doi: 10.1177/0115426506021003312.

18 **overestimate body weights at taller heights:** Shah, Sucher, and Hollenbeck. "Comparison of Ideal Body Weight Equations and Published Height-Weight Tables with Body Mass Index Tables for Healthy Adults in the United States."

19 **Hammond equation:** K. A. Hammond, "Dietary and Clinical Assessment." In L. Kathleen Mahan and Sylvia Escott-Stump, eds., *Krause's Food, Nutrition, & Diet Therapy,* 11th ed. (Philadelphia: Saunders, 2004), 353–79.

23 **Mifflin-St. Jeor equation:** M. D. Mifflin et al. "A New Predictive Equation for Resting Energy Expenditure in Healthy Individuals." *American Journal of Clinical Nutrition* 51, no. 2 (1990): 241–47. doi: 10.1093/ajcn/51.2.241.

25 **physical activity level (PAL) factor:** George A. Brooks, Nancy F. Butte, William M. Rand, et al. "Chronicle of the Institute of Medicine Physical Activity Recommendation: How a Physical Activity Recommendation Came to Be Among Dietary Recommendations." *American Journal of Clinical Nutrition* 79, no. 5 (2004): 921S–930S. doi: 10.1093/ajcn/79.5.921S.

25 **established by the Institute of Medicine:** Food and Nutrition Board, Institute of Medicine of the National Academies. *Dietary Reference Intakes for Energy, Carbohydrate, Fiber, Fat, Fatty Acids, Cholesterol, Protein, and Amino Acids* (Washington, DC: National Academies Press, 2005).

THE INTRICACIES OF BODY COMPOSITION

30 **gravitate toward sports that favor our current or potential body type:** Rebecca L. Carl, Miriam D. Johnson, Thomas J. Martin, and Council on Sports Medicine and Fitness. "Promotion of Healthy Weight-Control Practices in Young Athletes." *Pediatrics* 140, no. 3 (2017): e20171871. doi: 10.1542/peds.2017-1871.

33 **Body Fat Ranges for Health and Performance:** American Council on Exercise, https://www.acefitness.org/education-and-resources/lifestyle/tools-calculators/percent-body-fat-calculator; accessed August 4, 2021; Asker Jeukendrup and Michael Gleeson, *Sports Nutrition: An Introduction to Energy Production and Performance,* 2nd ed. (Champaign, IL: Human Kinetics, 2010). Available at https://us.humankinetics.com/blogs/excerpt/normal-ranges-of-body-weight-and-body-fat.

34 **The University of Oregon recently announced that coaches may no longer subject athletes to body composition measurements:** Ken Goe, "Oregon Ducks Athletic Programs No Longer Can Monitor Athletes' Weight, Body Fat Percentage," December 2, 2021. https://www.oregonlive.com/ducks/2021/12/oregon-ducks-athletic-programs-no-longer-can-monitor-athletes-weight-body-fat-percentage.html; accessed January 10, 2022.

STOPPING THE SWIRL AND SEEKING BODY POSITIVITY

38 **and bikini bottoms:** International Handball Federation. *IX. Rules of the Game, July 8, 2014.* https://www.ihf.info/sites/default/files/2019-05/0_09%20-%20Rules%20of%20the%20Game%20%28Beach%20Handball%29_GB.pdf; accessed July 30, 2021.

38 **wear shorts instead:** Jenny Gross, "Women's Handball Players Are Fined for Rejecting Bikini Uniforms." *New York Times*, July 20, 2021. www.nytimes.com/2021/07/20/sports/norway-beach-handball-team.html, accessed July 30, 2021.

39 **a pervasive dissatisfaction with one's body:** Joel R. Grossbard, Clayton Neighbors, and Mary E. Larimer. "Perceived Norms for Thinness and Muscularity Among College Students: What Do Men and Women Really Want?" *Eating Behaviors* 12, no. 3 (2011): 192–99. doi: 10.1016/j.eatbeh.2011.04.005.

39 **disenchantment with one's body begins as early as elementary school:** Lenka H. Shriver, Amanda W. Harrist, Melanie Page, et al. "Differences in Body Esteem by Weight Status, Gender, and Physical Activity

Among Young Elementary School-Aged Children." *Body Image* 10, no. 1 (2013): 78–84. doi: 10.1016 /j.bodyim.2012.10.005.

39 **stronger desire to *lose* weight:** Marita P. McCabe and Lina A. Ricciardelli. "Body Image Dissatisfaction Among Males Across the Lifespan: A Review of Past Literature." *Journal of Psychosomatic Research* 56, no. 6 (2004): 675-85. doi: 10.1016/S0022-3999(03)00129-6.

39 **from childhood to young womanhood:** Michaela M. Bucchianeri, Aimee J. Arikian, Peter J. Hannan, et al. "Body Dissatisfaction from Adolescence to Young Adulthood: Findings from a 10-Year Longitudinal Study." *Body Image* 10, no. 1 (2013): 1–7. doi: 10.1016/j. bodyim.2012.09.001.

39 **underweight women still see themselves as heavier than they really are:** Mona M. Voges, Claire-Marie Giabbiconi, Benjamin Schöne, et al. "Gender Differences in Body Evaluation: Do Men Show More Self-Serving Double Standards Than Women?" *Frontiers in Psychology* 10: 544. doi: 10.3389/fpsyg .2019.00544.

40 **rather than as "coaching issues":** J. Sundgot-Borgen and M. K. Torstveit. "Aspects of Disordered Eating Continuum in Elite High-Intensity Sports." *Scandinavian Journal of Medicine & Science in Sports* 20, suppl. 2 (2010): 112–21. doi: 10.1111/j.1600-0838.2010.01190.x.

AN INTRODUCTION TO ENERGY AND THE NUTRIENTS THAT MOVE US

48 **measly 17 grams or less:** NCHS, National Health and Nutrition Examination Survey, and U.S. Department of Agriculture, Agriculture Research Service. Beltsville Human Nutrition Research Center, Food Surveys Research Group, *What We Eat in America*. See Appendix I, National Health and Nutrition Examination Survey (NHANES). www.cdc.gov/nchs/data/hus/2019/024-508.pdf, accessed July 8, 2021.

48 **Higher fiber intake is linked to lower body weight:** Yunsheng Ma, Barbara C. Olendzki, Jinsong Wang, et al. "Single-Component Versus Multicomponent Dietary Goals for the Metabolic Syndrome: A Randomized Trial." *Annals of Internal Medicine* 162, no. 4 (2015): 248–57. doi: 10.7326/M14-0611.

54 **The DV for protein is 50 g/day:** "Daily Value and Percent Daily Value: Changes on the New Nutrition and Supplement Facts Labels." https://www.fda.gov/media/135301/download, accessed July 13, 2021.

55 **initiated by training:** D. Travis Thomas, Kelly Anne Erdman, and Louise M. Burke. "Position of the Academy of Nutrition and Dietetics, Dietitians of Canada, and the American College of Sports Medicine: Nutrition and Athletic Performance." *Journal of the Academy of Nutrition and Dietetics* 116, no. 3 (2016): 501–28. doi: 10.1016/j.jand.2015.12.006.

60 **USDA's FoodData Central:** U.S. Department of Agriculture, Agricultural Research Service. FoodData Central, 2019. https://fdc.nal.usda.gov.

63 **receive some 32 percent of their daily caloric intake from fat:** Zhilei Shan, Colin D. Rehm, Gail Rogers, et al. "Trends in Dietary Carbohydrate, Protein, and Fat Intake and Diet Quality Among US Adults, 1999–2016." *JAMA* 322, no. 12 (2019): 1178–87. doi:10.1001/jama.2019.13771.

63 **total calories from fat (27 percent versus 30 percent):** Kristen E. Gerlach, Harold W. Burton, Joan M. Dorn, et al. "Fat Intake and Injury in Female Runners." *Journal of the International Society of Sports Nutrition* 5, no. 1 (2008): 1. doi: 10.1186/1550-2783-5-1.

65 **published data suggest:** Karen Mumme and Welma Stonehouse. "Effects of Medium-Chain Triglycerides on Weight Loss and Body Composition: A Meta-Analysis of Randomized Controlled Trials." *Journal of the Academy of Nutrition and Dietetics* 115, no. 2 (2015): 249–63. doi: 10.1016/j.jand.2014.10.022.

66 **less than 10 percent of daily calories from saturated fat:** U.S. Department of Agriculture and U.S. Department of Health and Human Services. *Dietary Guidelines for Americans, 2020–2025,* 9th ed. December 2020. Available at DietaryGuidelines.gov.

69 **Micronutrients and the Foods to Choose:** U.S. Department of Health and Human Services. (2021). *Dietary Supplement Fact Sheets.* National Institutes of Health Office of Dietary Supplements. https://ods.od .nih.gov/factsheets/list-all/.

69 **How Much Is Needed Each Day:** American College of Obstetricians and Gynecologists. "Nutrition During Pregnancy: FAQs." https://www.acog.org/womens-health/faqs/nutrition-during-pregnancy; accessed September 10, 2021.

74 **the vegetables most frequently consumed in the United States:** Economic Research Service, U.S. Department of Agriculture. "Potatoes and Tomatoes Are the Most Commonly Consumed Vegetables." 2019. https://www.ers.usda.gov/data-products/chart-gallery/gallery/chart-detail/?chartId=58340; accessed September 6, 2021.

74 **take one or more supplements daily:** Elizabeth D. Kantor, Colin D. Rehm, Mengmeng Du, et al. "Trends in Dietary Supplement Use Among US Adults from 1999–2012." *JAMA* 316, no.14 (2016): 1464–74. doi: 10.1001/jama.2016.14403.

74 **Roughly 65 percent of female collegiate varsity athletes report consuming supplements:** Nancie H. Herbold, Bridget K. Visconti, Susan Frates, and Linda Bandini. "Traditional and Nontraditional Supplement Use by Collegiate Female Varsity Athletes." *International Journal of Sport Nutrition and Exercise Metabolism* 14, no. 5 (2004): 586–93. doi: 10.1123/ijsnem.14.5.586.

74 **vitamin C, iron, calcium, and magnesium:** Michelle T. Barrack, Mark Muster, Jennifer Nguyen, et al. 2021. "An Investigation of Habitual Dietary Supplement Use Among 557 NCAA Division I Athletes." *Journal of the American College of Nutrition* 39, no. 7 (2020): 619–27. doi: 10.1080/07315724.2020.1713247.

77 **Creatine Monohydrate:** Thomas W. Buford, Richard B. Kreider, Jeffrey R. Stout, et al. "International Society of Sports Nutrition Position Stand: Creatine Supplementation and Exercise." *Journal of the International Society of Sports Nutrition* 4 (2007): 6. doi: 10.1186/1550-2783-4-6.

77 **with minimal effects on body composition:** Joan M. Eckerson. "Creatine as an Ergogenic Aid for Female Athletes." *Strength and Conditioning Journal* 38, no. 2 (2016): 14–23. doi: 10.1519/SSC .0000000000000208.

77 **antidepressant effects:** Kyoon Lyoo, Sujung Yoon, Tae-Suk Kim, et al. "A Randomized, Double-Blind Placebo-Controlled Trial of Oral Creatine Monohydrate Augmentation for Enhanced Response to a Selective Serotonin Reuptake Inhibitor in Women with Major Depressive Disorder." *American Journal of Psychiatry* 169, no. 9 (2012): 937–45. doi: 10.1176/appi.ajp.2012.12010009.

77 **of particular importance during menses, pregnancy, postpartum, pre- and postmenopause:** Abbie E. Smith-Ryan, Hannah E. Cabre, Joan M. Eckerson, and Darren G. Candow. "Creatine Supplementation in Women's Health: A Lifespan Perspective." *Nutrients* 13, no. 3 (2021): 877. doi: 10.3390/ nu13030877.

78 **prolong moderate exercise performance:** Karen D. Mittleman, Matthew R. Ricci, and Stephen J. Bailey. "Branched-Chain Amino Acids Prolong Exercise During Heat Stress in Men and Women." *Medicine & Science in Sports & Exercise* 30, no.1 (1998): 83–91. doi: 10.1097/00005768-199801000-00012.

THE HIGH SCHOOL AND COLLEGE YEARS

115 **across a variety of sports:** Neoklis A. Georgopoulos, Nikolaos D. Roupas, Anastasia Theodoropoulou, et al. "The Influence of Intensive Physical Training on Growth and Pubertal Development in Athletes." *Annals of the New York Academy of Sciences* 1205, no. 1 (2010): 39–44. doi: 10.1111/j.1749-6632.2010.05677.x.

116 **subjects who reported sleeping less gained more weight than those who reported sleeping more:** Sanjay R. Patel, Atul Malhotra, David P. White, et al. "Association Between Reduced Sleep and Weight Gain in Women." *American Journal of Epidemiology* 164, no. 10 (2006): 947–54. doi: 10.1093/aje/kwj280.

MOM ON THE RUN

141 **miscarriages:** March of Dimes, "Miscarriage," https://www.marchofdimes.org/complications/miscarriage.aspx; accessed August 20, 2021.

141 **end in miscarriage:** Carla Dugas and Valori H. Slane. *"Miscarriage."* In StatPearls (Treasure Island, FL: StatPearls Publishing, 2022). https://www.ncbi.nlm.nih.gov/books/NBK532992/.

143 **Recommendations for Weight Gain During Pregnancy:** Institute of Medicine and National Research Council. *Weight Gain During Pregnancy: Reexamining the Guidelines* (Washington, DC: National Academies Press, 2009). doi: 10.17226/12584.

144 **Estimated Calorie Needs During Pregnancy and Lactation:** U.S. Department of Agriculture and U.S. Department of Health and Human Services. *Dietary Guidelines for Americans, 2020–2025,* 9th ed. December 2020, 111–12. https://www.dietaryguidelines.gov/sites/default/files/2020-12/Dietary_Guidelines_for_Americans_2020-2025.pdf.

144 **Estimated changes in daily calorie needs:** Institute of Medicine. *Dietary Reference Intakes for Energy, Carbohydrate, Fiber, Fat, Fatty Acids, Cholesterol, Protein, and Amino Acids* (Washington, DC: National Academies Press; 2005).

151 **accounting for the energy requirements of exercise:** Kathryn G. Dewey, Cheryl A. Lovelady, Laurie A. Nommsen-Rivers, et al. "A Randomized Study of the Effects of Aerobic Exercise by Lactating Women on Breast-Milk Volume and Composition." *New England Journal of Medicine* 330, no. 7 (1994): 449–53. doi: 10.1056/NEJM199402173300701.

154 **Dr. Lauren Borowski and her colleagues:** Lauren E. Borowski, Elizabeth I. Barchi, Julie S. Han, et al. "Musculoskeletal Considerations for Exercise and Sport: Before, During, and After Pregnancy." *Journal of the American Academy of Orthopaedic Surgeons* 29, no. 16 (2021): e805–e814. doi: 10.5435/JAAOS-D-21-00044.

157 *Sweat. Eat. Repeat.:* Pamela Nisevich Bede. *Sweat. Eat. Repeat.* (Boulder, CO: VeloPress, 2019).

158 **practice increasing:** International Food Information Council. *2020 Food & Health Survey.* https://foodinsight.org/wp-content/uploads/2020/06/IFIC-Food-and-Health-Survey-2020.pdf; accessed July 1, 2021.

160 **an increase in levels of circulating free fatty acids:** Grant M. Tinsley and Paul M. La Bounty. "Effects of Intermittent Fasting on Body Composition and Clinical Health Markers in Humans." *Nutrition Reviews* 73, no. 10 (2015): 661–74. doi: 10.1093/nutrit/nuv041.

162 **Aird and colleagues:** T. P. Aird, R. W. Davies, and B. P. Carson. "Effects of Fasted vs Fed-State Exercise on Performance and Post-Exercise Metabolism: A Systematic Review and Meta-Analysis." *Scandinavian Journal of Medicine & Science in Sports* 28, no. 5: 1476–93. doi: 10.1111/sms.13054.

163 glycogen (restocking energy stores): Anne-Marie Lundsgaard, Andreas M. Fritzen, and Bente Kiens. "The Importance of Fatty Acids as Nutrients During Post-Exercise Recovery." *Nutrients* 12, no. 2 (2020): 280. doi: 10.3390/nu12020280.

164 24 percent of consumers: International Food Information Council. *2020 Food and Health Survey.*

164 National Health and Nutrition Examination Survey (NHANES): Craig M. Hales, Margaret D. Carroll, Cheryl D. Fryar, and Cynthia L. Ogden. "Prevalence of Obesity and Severe Obesity Among Adults: United States, 2017–2018." National Center for Health Statistics Data Brief No. 360, February 2020. https://www.cdc.gov/nchs/products/databriefs/db360.htm.

164 while protein intake is increasing: Jacqueline D. Wright and Chia-Yih Wang. "Trends in Intake of Energy and Macronutrients in Adults from 1999–2000 Through 2007–2008." National Center for Health Statistics Data Brief No. 49, November 2010: 1-8. https://www.cdc.gov/nchs/products/databriefs/db49.htm; Centers for Disease Control and Prevention. "Trends in Intake of Energy and Macronutrients—United States, 1971–2000." *Morbidity and Mortality Weekly Report* 53, no. 4 (2004): 80–82. https://www.cdc.gov/mmwr/preview/mmwrhtml/mm5304a3.htm; NCHS, National Health and Nutrition Examination Survey, and U.S. Department of Agriculture, Agriculture Research Service. Beltsville Human Nutrition Research Center, Food Surveys Research Group, *What We Eat in America.* See Appendix I, National Health and Nutrition Examination Survey (NHANES). https://www.cdc.gov/nchs/data/hus/2019/024-508.pdf; accessed July 8, 2021.

167 Stacy Sims says: Stacy T. Sims and Selene Yeager. *Roar.* (New York: Harmony/Rodale, 2016).

169 a ten-week pilot study: Caryn Zinn, Matthew Wood, Mikki Williden, et al. "Ketogenic Diet Benefits Body Composition and Well-Being but Not Performance in a Pilot Case Study of New Zealand Endurance Athletes." *Journal of the International Society of Sports Nutrition* 14 (2017): 22. doi: 10.1186/s12970-017-0180-0. https://jissn.biomedcentral.com/articles/10.1186/s12970-017-0180-0.

176 outputs of performance such as power, agility: D. Travis Thomas, Kelly Anne Erdman, and Louise M. Burke. "Nutrition and Athletic Performance." *Medicine & Science in Sports & Exercise* 48, no. 3 (2016): 543–68. doi: 10.1249/MSS.0000000000000852.

FUEL YOUR PERFORMANCE: BEFORE, DURING, AND AFTER FUELING STRATEGIES

189 Stacy Sims explains that in the AM: Noelle Tarr and Stefani Ruper. "Women Are Not Small Men, with Dr. Stacy Sims." *Well-Fed Women* podcast, episode 317, March 20, 2021.

189 kisspeptin: Víctor M. Navarro. "Metabolic Regulation of Kisspeptin—The Link Between Energy Balance and Reproduction." *Nature Reviews Endocrinology* 16, suppl. 1 (2020): 407–20. doi: 10.1038/s41574-020-0363-7.

189 Kisspeptin also plays: Víctor M. Navarro. "Metabolic Regulation of Kisspeptin—The Link Between Energy Balance and Reproduction."

198 The exercise-linked enhancement of muscle protein synthesis: José L. Areta, Louise M. Burke, Megan L. Ross, et al. "Timing and Distribution of Protein Ingestion During Prolonged Recovery from Resistance Exercise Alters Myofibrillar Protein Synthesis." *Journal of Physiology* 591, no. 9 (2013): 2319–31.

199 inclusive of plasma volume: D. Travis Thomas, Kelly Anne Erdman, and Louise M. Burke. "Nutrition and Athletic Performance." *Medicine & Science in Sports & Exercise* 48, no. 3 (2016): 543–68. doi: 10.1249/MSS.0000000000000852.

205 **an intake of 14 to 27 ounces:** Phillip Watson, David Nichols, and Philip Cordery. "Mouth Rinsing with a Carbohydrate Solution Does Not Influence Cycle Time Trial Performance in the Heat." *Applied Physiology, Nutrition, and Metabolism* 39, no. 9 (2014): 1064–69. doi: 10.1139/apnm-2013-0413.

THE IMPACT OF MENSTRUATION

212 **menstrual hormones have an impact on substrate availability:** Macy M. Helm, Graham R. McGinnis, and Arpita Basu. 2021. "Impact of Nutrition-Based Interventions on Athletic Performance During Menstrual Cycle Phases: A Review." *International Journal of Environmental Research and Public Health* 18, no. 12 (2021): 6294. doi: 10.3390/ijerph18126294.

214 **in the week preceding menstruation:** Stacy T. Sims and Selene Yeager. *Roar.* (New York: Harmony/Rodale, 2016).

215 **can help improve performance:** Feng-Hua Sun, Stephen Heung-Sang Wong, Shi-Hui Chen, and Tsz-Chun Poon. "Carbohydrate Electrolyte Solutions Enhance Endurance Capacity in Active Females." *Nutrients* 7, no. 5 (2015): 3739–50. doi: 10.3390/nu7053739.

215 **every 5 kilometers does the trick:** Zhaohuan Gui, Fenghua Sun, Gangyan Si, and Yajun Chen. "Effect of Protein and Carbohydrate Solutions on Running Performance and Cognitive Function in Female Recreational Runners." *PLoS One* 12, no. 10 (2017): e0185982. doi: 10.1371/journal.pone.0185982.

220 **likely impacts as many as 50 percent of female athletes:** M. J. De Souza, R. J. Toombs, J. L. Scheid, et al. "High Prevalence of Subtle and Severe Menstrual Disturbances in Exercising Women: Confirmation Using Daily Hormone Measures." *Human Reproduction* 25, no. 2 (2010): 491–503. doi: 10.1093/humrep/dep411.

FIRESIDE CHAT: WHEN EATING GOES AWRY

223 **malnourished or even starving populations:** Mary Jane De Souza and Nancy I. Williams. "Physiological Aspects and Clinical Sequelae of Energy Deficiency and Hypoestrogenism in Exercising Women." *Human Reproduction Update* 10, no. 5 (2004): 433–48. doi: 10.1093/humupd/dmh033.

224 **required by the body to maintain optimal health and performance:** Margo Mountjoy, Jorunn Sundgot-Borgen, Louise Burke, et al. "The IOC Consensus Statement: Beyond the Female Athlete Triad—Relative Energy Deficiency in Sport (RED-S)." *British Journal of Sports Medicine* 48, no. 7 (2014): 491–97. doi: 10.1136/bjsports-2014-093502.

224 **LEA underpins RED-S:** Margo Mountjoy, Jorunn Kaiander Sundgot-Borgen, Louise M. Burke, et al. "IOC Consensus Statement on Relative Energy Deficiency in Sport (RED-S): 2018 Update." *British Journal of Sports Medicine* 52, no. 11 (2018): 687–97. doi: 10.1136/bjsports-2018-099193.

224 **many health and performance consequences associated with RED-S:** Mountjoy, Sundgot-Borgen, Burke, et al. "IOC Consensus Statement on Relative Energy Deficiency in Sport (RED-S): 2018 Update."

226 **Nearly 6 percent of the female athletes who completed the survey had a clinical eating disorder:** Leigh A. Sears, Kathryn R. Tracy, and Nicole M. McBrier. "Self-Esteem, Body Image, Internalization, and Disordered Eating Among Female Athletes." *Athletic Training and Sports Health Care* 4, no. 1 (2012): 29–37.

227 **aesthetically judged, gravitational, and weight-class sports:** Kimberley R. Wells, Nikki A. Jeacocke, Renee Appaneal, et al. "The Australian Institute of Sport (AIS) and National Eating Disorders Collaboration

(NEDC) Position Statement on Disordered Eating in High Performance Sport." *British Journal of Sports Medicine* 54, no. 21 (2020): 1247–58. doi: 10.1136/bjsports-2019-101813.

227 **mirrors the global incidence of eating disorders:** Jon Arcelus, Alex J. Mitchell, Jackie Wales, and Søren Nielsen. "Mortality Rates in Patients with Anorexia Nervosa and Other Eating Disorders. A Meta-Analysis of 36 Studies." *Archives of General Psychiatry* 68, no. 7 (2011): 724–31. doi: 10.1001/archgenpsychiatry .2011.74.

227 **6 to 45 percent in female athletes:** Solfrid Bratland-Sanda and Jorunn Sundgot-Borgen. "Eating Disorders in Athletes: Overview of Prevalence, Risk Factors and Recommendations for Prevention and Treatment." *European Journal of Sport Science* 13, no. 5 (2013): 499–508. doi: 10.1080/17461391.2012.740504.

232 **(DSM-5):** American Psychiatric Association. *Diagnostic and Statistical Manual of Mental Disorders, Fifth Edition (DSM-5), 2013.* https://doi.org/10.1176/appi.books.9780890425596.

233 **Anorexia Nervosa (AN):** National Eating Disorder Association website. https://www.nationaleatingdis orders.org/learn/by-eating-disorder/anorexia; accessed November 7, 2021.

233 **Bulimia Nervosa (BN):** National Eating Disorder Association website. https://www.nationaleatingdisor ders.org/learn/by-eating-disorder/bulimia; accessed November 7, 2021.

233 **Binge Eating Disorder (BED):** National Eating Disorder Association website. https://www.nationale atingdisorders.org/learn/by-eating-disorder/bed; accessed November 7, 2021.

234 **Other Specified Feeding or Eating Disorder (OSFED); previously referred to as Eating Disorder Not Otherwise Specified (EDNOS):** National Eating Disorder Association website. https://www.nationale atingdisorders.org/learn/by-eating-disorder/osfed; accessed November 7, 2021.

INDEX